Trends in Organ Transplantation

Barbara A. Williams, RN, BSN, is a staff nurse in the cardiothoracic intensive care unit at Stanford Health Services, Stanford, CA. She was an assistant nurse manager for 7 years in the cardiothoracic intensive care unit at Stanford Health Services and she has over 20 years experience in intensive care nursing. Her areas of transplant expertise include caring for heart, lung, and heart-lung recipients. Williams received her BS degree in nursing with distinction from San Jose State University, California. Her certificate as a nurse anesthetist is from Westend University Hospital, Berlin, Germany.

She presents lectures on transplant issues nationally and internationally and has been nominated and accepted into the fifth edition of *Who's Who in American Nursing.* Williams has written and published many articles on transplant nursing care and issues. She is the coeditor and coauthor of the book *Organ Transplantation: A Manual for Nurses,* published in 1991 by Springer Publishing Company, New York.

Williams is a member of the International Heart and Lung Transplantation Society, the International Transplant Nurses Society, the American Association of Critical Care Nurses, and the American Heart Association. She is the founder of the International Transplant Nurses Society, Northern California Chapter, and has been president since 1994.

Doris M. Sandiford-Guttenbeil, RN, BSN, is a staff nurse at Stanford Health Services, Stanford, CA. Her professional career encompasses 30 years, 28 of them in critical care at Stanford. She has presented lectures on transplantation, left ventricular assist device, and critical-care transport; she has coedited a nursing textbook, *Organ Transplantation: A Manual for Nurses,* published in 1991 by Springer Publishing Company; and has authored various articles and nursing guidelines on transplantation.

Sandiford-Guttenbeil received her registered nurse diploma from Chicago Wesley Memorial Hospital School of Nursing and her bachelor of science degree in nursing from Northwestern University in Illinois. She is certified in intra-aortic balloon pump (IABP) and left ventricular assist device system (LVAS) and serves on the Adult Critical Care Transport Team.

Trends in Organ Transplantation

Barbara A. Helene Williams, RN, BSN
Doris M. Sandiford-Guttenbeil, RN, BSN
Editors

Springer Publishing Company

Springer Publishing Company, Inc.
536 Broadway
New York, NY 10012-3955

Cover design by Tom Yabut
Production Editor: Joyce Noulas

96 97 98 99 00 / 5 4 3 2 1

Library of Congress Cataloging-in-Publication Data

Trends in organ transplantation / Barbara A. Helene Williams, Doris M. Sandiford-Guttenbeil, editors.
p. cm.
Includes bibliographical references and index.
ISBN 0-8261-9150-9
1. Transplantation of organs, tissues, etc.—Nursing.
2. Transplantation of organs, tissues, etc.. I. Williams, Barbara A. Helene. II. Sandiford-Guttenbeil, Doris M. (Doris Mae)
RD129.8.T74 1996
617.9'5—dc20 95-24993
CIP

Printed in the United States of America

Any medical or therapeutic agent or procedure described in this book should be applied by the practitioner under appropriate supervision in accordance with professional standards of care and the unique circumstances of each situation. Medically qualified readers are advised to consult the instructions and information included in package inserts of each drug or therapeutic agent before administration, particularly when using new or infrequently used drugs.

This book is dedicated to the hopes, healing, and dreams
of all donors, recipients, and health care providers.

Hope is a risk that must be run.

Georges Bernanos
Last Essays, 1955

Healing is a matter of time,
but it is sometimes also a matter of opportunity.

Hippocrates
460–400 B.C.

The dream, alone, is of interest.
What is life, without a dream?

Edmond Rostand
La Princesse Lointaine, 1885

Contents

Contributors

Laura L. Adams, BS, received her degree from Old Dominion University in Norfolk, VA, and attended the Wharton School of Business at the University of Pennsylvania for postgraduate studies in the Certified Employee Specialist Program. She has worked exclusively in the health care benefits field and is presently senior manager of specialty contracting at Stanford Health Services and Lucile Salter Packard Children's Hospital in Stanford, CA. Adams was instrumental in developing the "Center of Excellence" proposals for tissue and organ transplantation programs in 1990.

Mark L. Barr, MD, is associate professor of surgery, codirector of cardiothoracic transplantation, and director of cardiothoracic surgical research at the University of Southern California School of Medicine in Los Angeles.

Stuart M. Busse-Henry, BS, has been the organ procurement coordinator for the Multi-Organ Transplant Center at Stanford, CA, since 1991. He received his degree in biology from Randolph-Macon College in Ashland, VA, and his surgical technician training at the University of Virginia, Charlottesville. Prior to coming to Stanford, Busse-Henry assisted with research, organ procurement, and donor management at the University of Virginia and the University of Chicago.

Paul Greig, MD, FRCS(C), is director of the gastrointestinal transplant programme at The Toronto Hospital, University of Toronto. He has recently published work on the topic of quality of life following liver transplant.

Angela Johns, RN, MPA, OCN, is the nurse manager of the bone marrow transplant unit at Stanford Health Services, CA, and has been at Stanford since 1986. She graduated form Methodist Hospital, Brooklyn, NY, received her bachelor of science degree in nursing from California State University, and acquired her master's of public administration from the University of

San Francisco in 1987. She has worked as a staff nurse and in nursing management in the areas of critical care, trauma, oncology, and bone marrow transplantation. She has lectured on these topics at Northern California hospitals.

Joyce K. Johnston, RN, BSN, CCRN, CCTC, received her BS degree in nursing in 1971 from Loma Linda University in Loma Linda, CA, and is currently the administrative director of the heart and lung transplant program at Loma Linda University Medical Center. She is a well-known lecturer/writer in her specialty area of neonatal nursing.

Christopher L. Knoppel, RN, BA, CPTC, has been a multi-organ transplant coordinator at Stanford Health Services, CA, since 1992. He graduated with a BA in nursing from the University of Örebro, Sweden, and he holds a bachelor of arts degree in health services administration from St. Mary's College in Moraga, CA. He has over 10 years' critical care experience and previously was a transplant coordinator at the California Transplant Donor Network.

Jacqueline Lever, RN, MSN, attended the Pittsburgh Hospital School of Nursing and received her MS degree in nursing from the University of Pittsburgh. She is currently working as a research nurse for the University of Pittsburgh School of Pharmacy. She is coauthor and lecturer on research involving immunosuppressants, particularly FK506, and presently is focusing on women's health issues in the area of transplantation.

Gary Levy, MD, FRCP(C), is director of the multi-organ transplant programme at The Toronto Hospital, University of Toronto. He heads a team of 30 physicians and surgeons at The Toronto Hospital and maintains an extensive program of transplantation research.

Helen Luikart, BS, MSN, is currently a clinical transplant coordinator and nurse educator in the Department of Cardiothoracic Surgery for the heart and lung transplant program at Stanford University Medical Center, CA. She holds a BS degree from the University of Southwestern Louisiana and an MSN degree from the University of California in San Francisco. She is an assistant clinical professor in the Department of Physiological Nursing at the University of California in San Francisco.

Janet Madill, RD, is senior transplant dietitian in the Nutrition Department at The Toronto Hospital. She has published several articles and has presented internationally on liver transplantation. She is the recipient of two awards: the Ross Clinical Dietetics Award in 1991 and the Clinic Nutrition Practice Based Research Award in 1993.

Sarah A. Martin, RN, MS, was a pediatric transplant coordinator caring for liver and intestine candidates and recipients at The University of Pittsburgh Medical Center when her chapter was written. Martin has worked as a pediatric critical care clinical nurse specialist and staff nurse. She is currently employed at The University of Chicago Hospitals as a staff nurse in the pediatric intensive care unit.

Gwendolyn Mayes, MMSC, CPTC, is a public health analyst with the Division of Organ Transplantation (DOT), United States Department of Health and Human Services. She serves as the project officer for the Organ Procurement and Transplantation Network and the Scientific Registry of Transplant Recipients who contract with the United Network for Organ Sharing. Mayes also serves as the project officer for the study entitled "Institutional Factors which Influence the Likelihood of Living-Related Kidney Transplant Operations," and spearheads initiatives related to the performance of the Organ Procurement Organization, transplant legislation, and practical applications of transplant policies. She also has experience as an educational director, senior transplant coordinator, and critical care physician's assistant, and has a background in bioethics studies.

Pam McFarlin, RN, MSN, has worked in health care for 23 years. Her experience includes positions as staff nurse on a medical/surgical floor, assistant manager of an inpatient oncology unit, home liaison nurse, and home health nurse. She is currently the program manager for Stanford Health Services' hospital-based Home Health Department, Stanford, CA. She is responsible for overseeing daily operations, budget, program development, and coordination and marketing. She received her BS degree in nursing and her MS degree in nursing from San Jose State University in California.

Randall E. Morris, MD, is director of the laboratory for transplantation immunology in the Department of Cardiothoracic Surgery at the Stanford University School of Medicine, CA. He studied biology and medicine at the Stanford University School of Medicine. He is on the editorial boards for *Transplantation, Transplantation Proceedings,* and the *Journal of Heart and Lung Transplantation,* and he is a councillor for the International Transplantation Society.

Sara J. Munk, RN, BSN, received her BSN from the University of Wisconsin in Madison. She has been at Stanford Health Services for 11 years and currently is the case manager for cardiothoracic surgery, heart and lung transplants, and multi-organ transplants.

Felicia A. Schenkel, RN, BS, CCTC, is the cardiothoracic transplant coordinator at the University of Southern California University Hospital. She has lectured nationally and internationally on living related lobar transplantation. She received her nursing and health care administration degrees at Quinnipiac College, Hamden, CT.

Leslie Siconolfi, RN, MSN, CCRN, is currently the case manager for transplant services at the University of Pittsburgh Medical Center in Pennsylvania. Leslie received her bachelor of science degree in nursing from Duke University in Durham, NC. She completed her MA degree in the cardiovascular clinical specialty program at the University of Pittsburgh. Previously, she was staff development instructor for critical care and postanesthesia recovery units and the clinical director of two liver and multiple organ transplant intensive care units. Leslie is known for her general expertise and lecturing in critical care and transplantation. She has 15 years of multidisciplinary critical care experience and is active in the International Transplant Nurses Society.

Vaughn A. Starnes, MD, is professor of surgery and chief of cardiothoracic surgery and transplantation at the University of Southern California School of Medicine.

Nancy L. Stitt, RN, BSN, CCRN, is the clinical nurse educator for the liver, renal, and pancreas transplant service at the University of Pittsburgh Medical Center in Pennsylvania. She is cofounder and president emeritus of the International Transplant Nurses Society founded in 1992, a professional nursing society created to address the multifaceted needs of nurses giving direct patient care to both pre- and post-transplant recipients.

D. Kathryn Tierney, RN, MSN, is an oncology clinical nurse specialist. She currently works at the Bone Marrow Transplant Program at Stanford Health Services, Stanford, CA. In 1980, she received a bachelor of science degree in nursing from the University of Wisconsin in Madison, and in 1989, received her master of science degree in nursing from the University of Pennsylvania. Her work in bone marrow transplantation began in 1980 at the University of Washington Hospital, Seattle.

Jane A. Waskerwitz, RN, MSN, is a multi-organ transplant coordinator at Stanford Health Services, Stanford, CA. She has been caring for patients with end-stage organ failure—mainly kidney, pancreas, and liver—since 1972. Prior to her present position, she spent 18 years at the University of Michigan, where she also received her undergraduate and graduate degrees.

Kathleen A. Witmer, RN, BSN, received a bachelor of science degree in nursing from Seattle University in 1984. After 6 years in the cardiovascular intensive care setting, she became procurement coordinator for the California Transplant Donor Network. Witmer began working at Stanford University Medical Center in 1992. Her current position combines both the clinical and the procurement roles in the care of heart, heart–lung, and lung transplant program.

Foreword by Bruce A. Reitz, MD

The dream of replacing diseased parts with healthy organs has existed since ancient times. We are fortunate to be living at a time when this has achieved reality, and transplanted vital organs sustain literally thousands of recipients in countries around the world. In 1994, in the United States alone, 20,000 patients received kidney, liver, heart, lung, or pancreas transplants. With the help of the modern medical practices described in this volume, the majority of these patients return to lives of good health, hope, and promise.

In order to have achieved these results, transplant teams everywhere have developed tremendous expertise in all phases of transplant management. The authors, all experienced in transplant care, give a very clear and complete description of the phases of the transplantation process. Together, they also demonstrate that teamwork has always been at the heart of the transplant process. Many individuals must work together to achieve the kinds of results described here. Nursing roles exist at every step of the process; and consistent, caring, expert nursing is crucial to successful outcomes.

Although the emphasis here is on the nursing aspects of the transplant process, the information is so comprehensive and well presented that all members of the transplant team can benefit, as well as patients and their families. The field continues to progress at such a breathtaking rate that, in just the last 4 years since these editors published their first book, new treatments and improved results have occurred. The contributors and editors are to be greatly commended for their efforts in producing this helpful text.

BRUCE A. REITZ, MD
Professor and Chairman
Department of Cardiothoracic Surgery
Stanford University Medical Center
Stanford, CA

Foreword by Connie R. Curran, EdD, RN, FAAN

As our country's health care expenditures approach 14% of the gross domestic product (GDP), health care reform became a national priority. The federal government, state governments, and employees (the three principal purchasers of health care) are all focused on reducing costs and assuring quality, and this focus applies to organ transplantation as well. Managed care is an approach that has been effective in lowering costs and yielding verifiable measures of quality of service.

The percentage of Americans participating in managed care plans will continue to increase, and this growth presents several unique challenges to those involved in organ transplantation because transplantation requires numerous human and material resources in prehospital evaluation, pretransplant care, transplantation specialists and staff, and posttransplant care. Because of these resource requirements, some managed care contracts are failing to provide coverage for certain high-risk, high-cost procedures. It will become increasingly difficult for hospitals to secure organ transplant contracts. To secure these contracts, hospitals will have to prove that their programs are cost-effective and meet very stringent outcome criteria.

The ethical issues surrounding organ transplantation are as complex as the economic issues. The United States has not developed national guidelines, as some countries have. When Oregon attempted to ration health care services, it saw strong positive and negative public reaction. Some groups have proposed denying organ transplants to individuals whose lifestyles, i.e., smoking, drinking, etc., have contributed to their organ disease.

The challenges and opportunities in organ transplantation will undoubtedly increase. The skills of competent, caring, and cost-conscious health care professionals are essential to moving forward in this important arena. This book is a valuable resource for nurses and other health professionals seeking an in-depth understanding of the complex issues surrounding organ transplantation.

CONNIE R. CURRAN, EdD, RN, FAAN
Vice Chairman, APM, Inc.

Preface

As we enter the 21st century, health care professionals will play key roles in making changes and meeting new challenges. Health care is in transition as it shifts from inpatient to outpatient care. In this transition, health care professionals will continue finding new ways to do things differently and more cost effectively. Nurses will find themselves in a unique position to contribute new models of economical and efficient health care delivery.

Our previous book, *Organ Transplantation: A Manual for Nurses,* also published by Springer Publishing Company, discussed the basic concepts of this field of nursing. *Trends in Organ Transplantation* gives health care professionals up-to-date information about what is new in organ transplantation. It answers some of the questions that organ recipients and their families ask nurses. In addition, *Trends in Organ Transplantation* addresses the impact of change in health care, including cost containment measures in the clinical setting, home care, and the application of clinical pathways. It discusses new immunosuppressive therapies, topics of special interest to women, and economics of transplantation and explores alternatives to transplantation.

We want to thank the many contributing authors who have enthusiastically written their chapters with the goal of sharing their expertise with their peers in the health care work place.

Acknowledgments

This book became a reality with the contributions from and cooperation of many people. I am deeply indebted and thankful to the authors who made this book real. Their devotion and intense efforts were inspirational and are much appreciated.

Donna Dowdney, PhD, deserves a special thank you for her editorial assistance and unfailing support.

Lois Manning did a great job in assisting, preparing, and completing the manuscript. I thank her for a project well done.

Barbara A. Williams

I would like to thank the contributors to this nursing textbook on organ transplantation. I appreciate their willingness to share their expertise with us.

Doris M. Sandiford-Guttenbeil

PART I

Impact of Changes in Nursing Care

1

ORGAN DONATION: A COLLABORATIVE COMMITMENT

Kathleen A. Witmer, R.N., B.S.N., C.P.T.C., and
Christopher L. Knoppel, R.N., B.A., C.P.T.C.

Every day, families choose life over death when they decide to donate a loved one's organs for the purpose of transplantation. As a result, thousands of lives each year are saved or enhanced thanks to altruism and a desire to make something good come from a personal tragedy.

Transplantation continues to evolve as an accepted treatment modality for patients suffering from end organ failure. Due to the advances in surgical techniques and in the field of immunosuppression, and public and professional support, the demand for all types of organ transplants has skyrocketed. The supply of organs suitable for transplantation, however, has remained relatively unchanged for the last 5 years, despite legislative and organized efforts. Alternative approaches to increase organ donation are currently being debated on both national and local levels. Financial incentives for donor families and presumed consent for donation are two controversial initiatives that have not gained widespread support. A nonprofit group called the Coalition on Donation has joined forces with the Ad Council to start a national education campaign in an effort to increase donor awareness. Their campaign slogan is, "Share Your Life, Share Your Decision."

With no clear solutions in the near future, health care professionals continue to struggle with criteria for organ donation, how to care for potential organ donor families, the declaration of brain death, and managing the donation process.

This chapter is an overview of the organ donation process. Discussion will encompass legislation that directly impacts professional and clinical practice, the current supply and demand of donor organs, reasons why organ donation may not occur, organ donor identification, understanding brain death declaration, meeting the critical needs of organ donor families, and recommendations for ensuring a timely and sensitive discussion about organ donation.

ORGAN DONATION AND THE LAW

Although legal and organizational developments over the last two decades have removed some of the major barriers to organ donation, it is imperative for health care professionals to have a working knowledge of the laws pertaining to the declaration of brain death and obtaining consent for organ donation. These laws provide the necessary foundation and guidance for practicing clinicians involved in the organ donation process.

The Uniform Anatomical Gift Act

The Uniform Anatomical Gift Act (UAGA) of 1968 remains the key piece of legislation supporting organ donation. This act made it legal to donate the organs of a deceased individual for transplantation and protected health care professionals from potential liability surrounding organ procurement. It is from this law that the use of organ donor cards originated, and it outlined the order of persons who can legally consent to donation.

The advent of life-support systems in the 1960s made organ donation and transplantation a reality. However, it was not until after Dr. Norman E. Shumway performed the first human heart transplant at Stanford University that the medical community in the United States began to tackle the issue of brain death. In 1968, an initial attempt was made to outline neurological criteria for the determination of death by the Ad Hoc Committee of the Harvard Medical School, but a uniform standard of death was not achieved until much later.

The Uniform Determination of Death Act

Finally, in 1981 the medical and legal communities reached a consensus on the definition of brain death. The Uniform Determination of Death Act (UDDA) provided that:

> An individual who has sustained either (1) irreversible cessation of circulatory and respiratory function, or (2) irreversible cessation of all functions of the entire brain, including the brain stem, is dead. A determination of death must be made in accordance with accepted medical standards. (President's Commission for the Study of Ethical Problems in Medicine and Biomedical and Behavioral Research, 1981)

The National Organ Transplant Act

In 1984, Congress passed The National Organ Transplant Act (NOTA) and began to regulate organ donation and transplantation. This act prohibited the purchase and sale of organs in the United States. It established the Organ Procurement and Transplantation Network (OPTN), which contracted with The United Network for Organ Sharing (UNOS) to manage organ distribution and establish a scientific registry. The national waiting list is maintained by UNOS. Locally, Organ Procurement Organizations (OPO) coordinate the day-to-day activities in the donation and transplantation process. They are the link between the donor hospitals, transplant centers, and UNOS.

The Omnibus Reconciliation Act

Further mandates in 1986 required hospitals receiving Medicare and Medicaid funding to establish written protocols for potential donor identification and procedures designed to ensure that families of potential donors be offered the option of donation. This is commonly referred to as "Required Request Legislation." Hospitals are required by the Joint Commission for the Accreditation of Health Organizations to show documented compliance with this legislation.

PUBLIC AND PROFESSIONAL SUPPORT FOR ORGAN DONATION

Despite the lack of increase of available donors, public and professional support for organ donation and transplantation continues to be strong.

Nearly 9 out of 10 Americans support the concept of organ donation (The Gallup Organization, 1993). Eighty-four percent of Americans strongly approve of organ donation, and 74% would want to donate their own organs in the event of their death (The Gallup Organization, 1990).

Professional support for donation is also strong. Health care professionals likewise have indicated overwhelming support for organ donation. More than 90% of nurses and physicians agree with organ donation and would agree to being donors themselves (Partnership for Organ Donation [POD], 1991). In spite of this overwhelming support, the number of organ donors in the United States each year has remained stagnant while the demand continues to escalate.

CURRENT DEMAND FOR TRANSPLANTATION

Organ transplantation is successful. (See Table 1.1 for survival rates.) The field of transplantation has evolved from speculation and research to providing a therapeutic and accepted medical therapy to thousands of patients suffering from end organ failure. In most cases, transplantation is the treatment of choice for end organ failure.

By the fall of 1994, over 36,000 patients were waiting for an organ transplant and holding on to the hope of improving their quality of life. Thousands of lives are lost each year that could be saved through transplantation. One-third of the adults and one-half of the children waiting in the United States will not survive to transplantation (UNOS, 1994). The

TABLE 1.1 One-Year Graft Survival Rates

Heart	82%
Heart-lung	66%
Lung	69%
Liver	73%
Pancreas*	51%
Simultaneous pancreas-kidney*	76%
Kidney-cadaveric	84%
Kidney-living donor	95%

Note. Adapted from *Organ Procurement Transplantation Network Annual Report: Graft and Patient Survival Rates,* by the United Network for Organ Sharing (UNOS), 1994.
*"Analysis of United States pancreas transplant registry data," by K. C. Moudry-Munns, A. Gruessner, & D. E. R. Sutherland, *Journal of Transplant Coordination, 4,* 18–22.

disparity between supply and demand is enormous and continues to plague the transplant community.

The current situation without intervention will get worse. With a 15% annual increase in the number of individuals waiting for an organ transplant, it is predicted that over 65,000 patients will be waiting by the end of the year 2000 (see Figure 1.1).

CURRENT SUPPLY OF DONOR ORGANS

Over the last 5 years, the actual number of organ donors has remained around 4,500 per year. According to conservative estimates, the potential donor pool is somewhere between 12,000 and 15,000 annually (The Partnership for Organ Donation, 1991). Variations between estimates are directly related to the criteria used to determine which potential donors were medically suitable. At best, only one-third of the potential donor pool is being realized.

ORGAN DONOR CRITERIA

In practice, there is wide variation in the donor selection criteria that directly impacts organ procurement and the number of transplants performed at any given center. The general organ donor criteria include the following (California Transplant Donor Network, 1994):

- Intact circulation
- No history of malignancies except primary brain tumors
- No transmissible infectious diseases
- No high-risk groups for AIDS
- Brain death established
- Consent from next-of-kin and coroner

Age limits for donors vary across the country as transplant centers work to expand their donor criteria in order to save more lives through transplantation. The current age range for organ donation is between newborn and 70 years; however, organs have been successfully transplanted from donors over 70 years of age.

The majority of organ donors being referred to Organ Procurement Organizations today are patients who have died as a result of cerebral vascular accidents or other medical causes, rather than patients who have

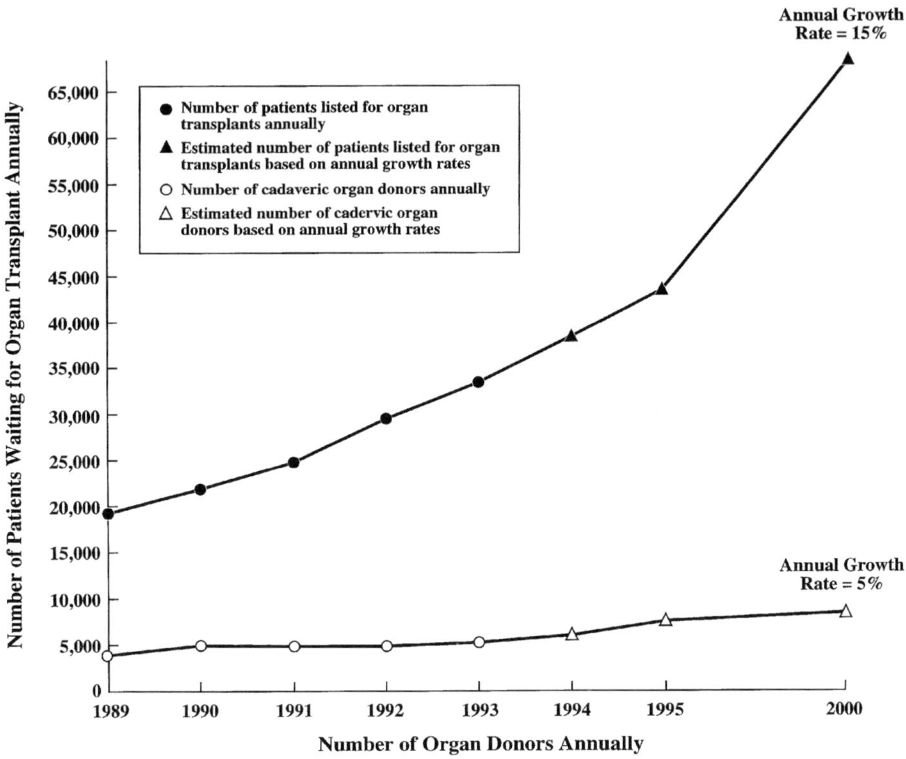

FIGURE 1.1 Supply and demand imbalance. From *Solving the Organ Donor Shortage,* by the Partnership for Organ Donation, Inc., 1991, and *Organ Procurement Transplantations Network annual report: Graft and patient survival rates,* by the United Network for Organ Sharing, 1994. Adapted with permission of the authors.

died from trauma. According to the Department of Transportation, recent vehicle safety laws (i.e., mandatory seat belts, air bags, helmet laws, and stiffer penalties for drunken driving) have decreased the number of motor vehicle fatalities by approximately 20% (Lombardo, 1994).

COMMON REASONS WHY DONATION MAY NOT OCCUR

Understanding where breakdowns in the donation process can occur may assist health care professionals to develop strategies that can improve the donation process in their own facilities. Lost opportunities may also identify the need for additional staff education. According to a survey of the OPO directors, there are three major reasons why donation does not occur.

Families Decline to Donate

The majority of donors are lost when families decline to donate. More than one-third of the families approached decline the option of organ donation (Association of Organ Procurement Agencies & Corporate Decisions, Inc., 1989; The Partnership for Organ Donation, Inc., 1991). Families may decline for various reasons; however, it is important to make sure that each family has been afforded a sensitive and timely approach. Even those families that decline to donate appreciate having been presented with the option.

Families not Presented With the Option to Donate

Approximately 17% of families are never approached about donation following brain death despite the required request laws established to prevent this very situation (Association of Organ Procurement & Corporate Decisions, Inc., 1989). If there is any perceived conflict of interest regarding patient care or medical treatment, physicians and nurses may opt out of the discussion with the family. Medical teams are trained to save lives. The greatest reluctance in talking with families stems from the fear of interfering with their grief or burdening them with yet one more request. Health care providers want to protect the family, but in doing so, they eliminate the possibility of the family's participating in an experience that may actually help and comfort them in their grief (The Partnership of Organ Donation, Inc., 1991).

Brain Death Unrecognized or Undeclared

In more than 12% of potential donors, brain death is unrecognized or undeclared (Association of Organ Procurement Agencies & Corporate Decisions, Inc., 1989). In order for organ donation to take place, brain death must be established. Etiologies commonly leading to brain death might include the following:

- Head trauma (motor vehicle accident, gunshot wound, suicide, homicide, etc.)
- Subarachnoid hemorrhage (CVA, arteriovenous malformation, aneurysm, etc.)

- Primary brain tumor
- Cerebral anoxia (drug overdose, near drowning, hanging, etc.) (California Transplant Donor Network, 1994, pp. 3–9)

Physicians may prefer to avoid brain death declaration and the explanation of an emotionally charged subject with grieving families. Health care providers sometimes fear that the diagnosis of brain death may burden the family. Those who do not clearly understand brain death are ambivalent about discussing it with families.

UNDERSTANDING BRAIN DEATH

Brain death is a medical diagnosis. Today, there still exists confusion surrounding brain death and brain death declaration for three basic reasons:

1. Although almost all states recognize that an individual may die from brain death, the actual language used in these laws varies from state to state.

2. States have outlined the procedures for declaring brain death to be followed by institutions and physicians based on accepted medical standards in their respective communities. It is important to recognize that these standards differ from state to state.

3. Brain death declaration is left to the discretion of the attending physician(s). The physician(s), in compliance with state regulations and independent of any transplant team, must perform a clinical examination. Confirmatory tests (EEG, cerebral blood-flow study, etc.) may be performed at the discretion of the physician(s) before a patient is declared brain-dead.

Brain Death: Criteria for Diagnosis

Criteria for brain death are broken down into the categories of absolute and optional. Absolute criteria include the following:

- Known cause of condition
- Absence of hypothermia (temperature greater than 32.2°C)
- Absence of CNS depressants
- Absence of cranial reflexes
- Absence of spontaneous respirations
- Cerebral unresponsiveness

Optional criteria include:

- Electrocerebral silence (EEG)
- Absence of cerebral perfusion (cerebral arteriogram, blood flow study)
- Absence of evoked potentials (President's Commission, 1981, pp. 2184–2187)

Health care professionals who are neither knowledgeable about legal criteria nor accurate in their concepts of brain death are ill prepared to discuss this issue with potential donor families (Younger, Landefeld, Coulton, Juknialis, & Leary, 1989). It is important for clinicians working in the critical care setting to be familiar with federal and state laws pertaining to the declaration of brain death. In addition, health care professionals need to consult the written protocols that address these issues as well as policies for donor identification and donor referral in their respective hospitals. A working knowledge of these laws will enable nurses to support families who find themselves presented with the option of donation and thus to minimize the number of lost opportunities.

FAMILY NEEDS IN ORGAN DONATION

The families of critically ill patients have specific needs the minute their loved ones are admitted to the intensive care unit. The admission represents a crisis situation for both patients and families. With severe head-injured patients, the families are dealing with life-threatening situations. They are experiencing an "extreme sense of helplessness, disruption, loss, fear, and anxiety" (Artinian, 1991, pp. 269–275). Nursing research has consistently shown that families in the critical care setting have identified their primary needs in the categories of assurance, proximity, and information (Leske, 1991).

Assurance

Reassurance and support are essential to a family suddenly faced with multiple decisions regarding medical treatment, personal business, and financial issues. The focus of family members will be the patient's survival and/or quality of life. Factors that affect their decision-making ability include coping skills, relationships, information, uncertain outcomes, environment, and emotions (Mirr, 1991).

Critical care nurses share the responsibility to care for families as well as patients (Mirr, 1991). Nursing interventions for family support should always be incorporated early in the care of potential organ donors such as patients with severe head injuries. Without early interventions, it becomes increasingly difficult to reassure and support a family if their loved one's condition should deteriorate. Additional sources of support for families in crisis often include social workers, chaplains, and family friends. These sources should be utilized whenever possible.

Cultural diversity among families must also be accommodated to reassure them that their loved ones are receiving the very best care available. It is important that the health care team be sensitive to families' needs with respect to culture.

Proximity

Families need frequent contact with the patient and a compassionate nursing staff (Pelletier, 1993). Access to their loved one will allow them to see that every effort is being made to care for their family member. It will also help them begin to process the information that they are receiving from the health care team regarding the patient's prognosis. The visiting hours in critical care units frequently limit the family's access to their loved one. Permission to visit frequently and to participate in patient care is important in the support of potential donor families.

Information

The greatest need experienced by families in the critical care setting is that of information. Families will need information on the patient's prognosis, routines and care, the critical care environment, etc. It is important to update the family frequently. Communication should be regular, honest, and consistent among the health care team, again to assure the family that their loved one is receiving the best care possible. Families may be asked to assimilate a great deal of information in a very short period of time. It may only be a matter of days following a sudden and traumatic injury before a family is informed of a poor prognosis or that their loved one is brain-dead. It is the responsibility of the health care team—and often it falls to the nurses—to clarify and reinforce medical information. How well nurses and physicians understand brain death and the procedures to declare brain death will determine their ability to explain it to a grieving family (Chabalewski & Norris, 1994).

While most people believe that death occurs when the heart stops and a person stops breathing, that is not the case with brain death. This is a concept with which most families are not familiar. The appearance of life continues as the ventilator simulates breathing and the heart beat appears on the monitor. The patient's skin feels warm and looks pink. For all intents and purposes, it appears that the patient is merely sleeping.

Brain Death = Death. Using the term "brain death" rather than death can be confusing to families. Because families may be unfamiliar with the concept of brain death, the meaning may be unclear and they may question the implication of such a term. In their minds, it may imply that the brain and not the patient has died. The media regularly report that patients who have been declared brain dead later "die" when "life support" is discontinued. Health care professionals also use terminology that implies that the patient dies twice (Younger et al., 1989).

Again, brain death is a medical diagnosis and not a family decision. Health care providers must be factual in their explanations about the cause of death and about which systems are working and which ones are not. It is helpful to explain the use of machines and medications that support vital organ function and to avoid hospital jargon. Instead, use clear and simple language to facilitate understanding. Reinforce the fact that the situation is irreversible and allow the family time to process this information. Health care professionals should avoid mixed messages and confusing terminology. Be careful to substitute "artificial support" for "life support" or "breathing machine" in the care of a brain-dead patient.

The clarity of information is important for a number of reasons. Lack of clarity leaves health care professionals uncomfortable in managing patients and may negatively influence their ability to support families or offer the option of donation when appropriate. Explanations should be repeated as often as necessary until the family understands that their loved one has died. "The family must clearly understand that the patient is dead before being offered the option of organ donation" (Chabalewski & Norris, 1994, pp. 28–33).

In the present era of sophisticated diagnostic and therapeutic technology, the most basic aspect of medicine is being neglected—communication. With the medical advances in this century and the variety of treatment options available, there must be effective communication if families are to make appropriate decisions.

RECOMMENDATIONS FOR THE ORGAN DONATION PROCESS

Talking to a family about organ donation can be a difficult and emotional process. It is not uncommon for families to be approached about donation before the appropriate time. Disasters occur when the family is presented with the donation option in the emergency room or the ICU waiting room before they have had access to their loved one or before they have been informed of the prognosis. Presenting the diagnosis of brain death and a request for organ donation in the same breath can create emotional turmoil for a family that has not yet accepted the death of their loved one. Families process information at their own pace. Every family is different. It is important to assess the family situation and carefully plan an individualized approach before engaging in a conversation about donation. The following steps are recommended to ensure a timely and sensitive approach to all families regarding the option for donation.

Step 1: Potential Donor Identification

The donation process begins when a member of the medical team recognizes that a patient has suffered a severe brain injury that has resulted or soon will result in brain death. The medical staff conducts clinical examinations to determine the neurological status of the patient.

Step 2: Referral to the Organ Procurement Organization

Successful organ donation requires that the nurse or physician identify potential donors and refer them as early as possible to the local Organ Procurement Organization (OPO). The OPO should be notified about all potential donors. All deaths may represent a potential donation and should be referred. Early referrals enable the OPO staff to give adequate evaluation to each situation and each opportunity for donation. The OPO will thoroughly evaluate each referral to determine medical suitability *before* talking with the family of a potential donor. They are also trained to assist the medical team with medical management of the brain-dead patient. This includes fluid and ventilatory management as well as diagnostic and laboratory tests necessary to evaluate each organ system.

Step 3: Explanation of Brain Death

Brain death is a concept that is unfamiliar to most families. They often require extra time and support while attempting to understand that their loved one has died. The diagnosis of brain death must be clearly communicated to the family by the physician, and explanations should be repeated as often as necessary until the family verbalizes understanding. Physicians must avoid the subject of organ donation until the family has acknowledged the death. Brain death should be discussed first, and the option of donation presented in a separate conversation (POD, 1991).

Step 4: Presenting the Donation Option

The request for donation should never be made until the family has moved beyond the initial shock of death and is emotionally ready to consider donation. When the family has acknowledged the death of their loved one, a health care professional presents the option of organ donation to the family or next-of-kin. The person with the most experience, expertise, and rapport with the family may be in the best position to approach them about organ donation. This may be the physician, the nurse, the OPO coordinator, the social worker, or any combination of health care professionals.

OPO coordinators are trained in bereavement counseling and in offering families the donation option. They can provide accurate information regarding the donation process and will work with the nursing staff to make sure that the family makes an informed decision. If there are religious or cultural considerations, the OPO staff will address these. The family discussion in the donation process does not involve pressure or coercion. Families are informed of their right to donate and their options regarding organ donation and are encouraged to take their time in making whatever decision is best for them.

Figure 1.2 is an algorithm that represents an overview of the recommended donation process.

IMPACT OF DONATION ON FAMILIES

Donor families benefit from having participated in organ donation. They find comfort in knowing that something positive has resulted from their loss. Eighty-nine percent of donor families have said that they would donate again, while 79% say that organ donation helped them in their grieving process (Prottas & Batten, 1986). By not offering the option of donation, health care providers make the decision for the family *not* to donate (Chabalewski & Norris, 1994). (See Table 1.2.)

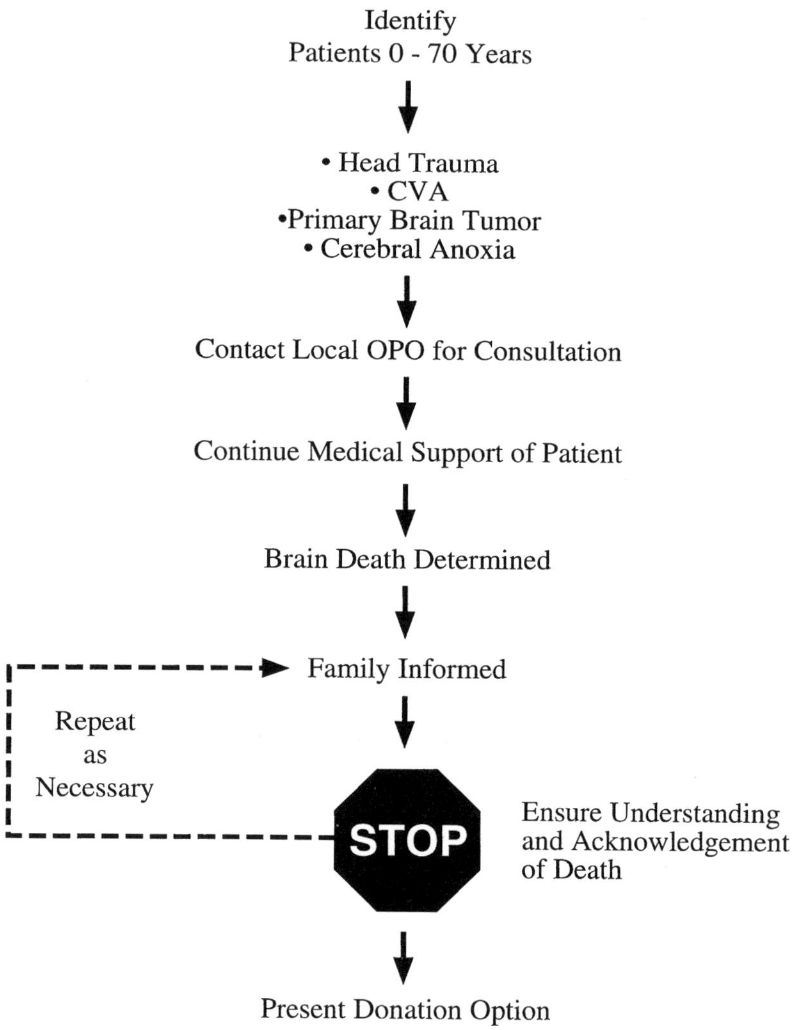

FIGURE 1.2 The donation process: an overview. From personal communication with P. Weber, August 1994, and from California Transplant Donor Network, 1991. Adapted by permission.

THE COLLABORATIVE COMMITMENT

The lack of knowledge regarding brain-death declaration among health care professionals may be directly related to their personal and profes-

TABLE 1.2 Organ Donation: It's a Legal Right

"The opportunity to donate their organs and tissues is a legal right guaranteed to all adult U.S. citizens through legislation adopted in some form by every state. The Uniform Anatomical Gift Act specifically recognizes this right and provides that when the individual's intent isn't known, the next-of-kin, in a defined order of priority, will make this decision.

With the intense stress and grief that follows a death—especially an unexpected or untimely one—family members are unlikely to think about organ and tissue donation on their own. But it can't be put off. Organs and tissues must be recovered within a limited time; otherwise a potentially life-saving gift will be irretrievably lost. That's why the law wisely shifts the responsibility for raising the subject of donation from the grief-stricken family to the health care professional.

As a patient and family advocate, you have a special duty to ensure that this right to choose is protected and carried out. The family members will make the decision, but if the option is never offered, the decision has been made for them. And that's illegal."

Note. From "The Gift of Life: Talking to Families about Organ and Tissue Donation," by F. Chabalewski & M. K. G. Norris, *American Journal of Nursing, 94,* 28–33.

sional experience with death and their degree of exposure to brain-dead patients. Differences in attitudes toward organ donation, required request laws, the effects of teaching programs, and variations in personal concepts of death contribute to the confusion that exists among nurses and physicians. The public looks to health care professionals to play a leadership role in clarifying the issues surrounding death. In order to meet the challenge, health care professionals must first clarify their own thinking (Younger et al., 1989).

The unexpected death of a family member combined with the consideration of donation and the logistics involved creates specific needs for the family that require attention from health care providers. Hospitals and health care professionals have a responsibility to incorporate organ donation into the care that they provide to all patients and their families. The issues of brain death, organ donation, and bereavement are complex. Families benefit from a collaborative effort on the part of all members of the health care team. These same physicians and nurses work side by side every day to save lives and comfort families. Their efforts are supported by social workers, chaplains, and other ancillary services. Regardless of the situation, they must work together to deliver quality care. It is the same teamwork that is needed to care for families faced with a sudden death and organ donation. In coordinating the care of potential donor families, the goals of the health care team should be accomplished in the following order:

- Meet the needs of the family
- Provide timely and accurate information
- Identify potential donor and refer to the local OPO
- Explain brain death and ensure understanding
- Support the family and allow them time to process information
- Present the donation option to the family

In closing, a successful donation process demands a collaborative effort among all health care professionals to impact the donation process and, more importantly, the care of the donor family. It is only through a collaborative commitment that acute care nurses, physicians, and allied health care professionals can impact how the donation option is presented to families and ultimately address the donor shortage.

REFERENCES

Ad Hoc Committee of the Harvard Medical School. (1984). A definition of irreversible coma. *Journal of the American Medical Association, 252,* 677–680.

Artinian, N. T. (1991). Strengthening nurse-family relationships in critical care. In J. S. Leske & J. M. Clochesy (Eds.), *AACN clinical issues in critical care nursing: Family interventions* (pp. 269–275). Philadelphia: J. B. Lippincott.

Association of Organ Procurement Agencies and Corporate Decisions, Inc. (1989). [Survey of Organ Procurement Organization Directors]. Unpublished raw data.

Batten, H. L., & Prottas, J. M. (1986). Kind strangers: The families of organ donors. *Health Affairs, 6,* 35–47.

California Transplant Donor Network. (Ed.) (1994, March). *Resource manual for organ and tissue donation* (pp. 3–9). (Available from California Transplant Donor Network, 55 Francisco Street, Suite 510, San Francisco, CA 94133-2115.)

California Transplant Donor Network. (1994, August). Phone interview with Phyllis Weber, R.N., Executive Director. San Francisco, CA.

Chabalewski, F., & Norris, M. K. G. (1994). The gift of life: Talking to families about organ and tissue donation. *American Journal of Nursing, 94,* 28–33.

The Gallup Organization, Inc. [survey conducted for the Partnership for Organ Donation]. (1990). *Americans and organ donation: Current attitudes and perceptions.* Boston: Author.

The Gallup Organization, Inc. [survey conducted for the Partnership for Organ Donation]. (1993). *The American public's attitudes toward organ donation and transplantation.* Boston: Author.

Leske, J. S. (1991). Overview of family needs after critical illness: From assessment to intervention. In J. S. Leske & J. M. Clochesy (Eds.), *AACN clinical issues in critical care nursing: Family interventions* (pp. 220–226). Philadelphia: J. B. Lippincott.

Lombardo, L. B. (1994, February). Trends in automobile deaths and injuries. In J. B. Braslow (Chair), *The potential donor pool: Selected trends and data.* Symposium conducted at the meeting Transplantation at the National Forefront, Washington, DC.

Mirr, M. P. (1991). Decisions made by family members of patients with severe head injury. In J. S. Leske & J. M. Clochesy (Eds.), *AACN clinical issues in critical care nursing: Family interventions* (pp. 242–251). Philadelphia: J. B. Lippincott.

Moudry-Munns, K. C., Gruessner, A., & Sutherland, D. E. R. (1994). Analysis of United States pancreas transplant registry data. *Journal of Transplant Coordination, 4,* 18–22.

The Partnership for Organ Donation, Inc. (1991). *Solving the organ donor shortage.* Boston: Author.

Pelletier, M. (1991). The organ donor family member's perception of stressful situations during the organ donation experience. *Journal of Advanced Nursing, 17,* 90–97.

Pelletier, M. (1993). The needs of family members of organ and tissue donors. *Heart & Lung, 22,* 151–157.

President's Commission for the Study of Ethical Problems in Medicine and Biomedical and Behavioral Research. (1981). Guidelines for the determination of death. *Journal of the American Medical Association, 246,* 2184–2187.

Prottas, J. M., & Batten, H. L. (1986). *Attitudes and incentives in organ procurement: Report to the Healthcare Financing Administration. Part 3. Giving families: Relatives of organ donors.* Washington, DC: Author.

United Network for Organ Sharing. (1994). *Organ Procurement Transplantation Network annual report: Graft and patient survival rates.* Richmond, VA: Author.

Younger, S. J., Landefeld, C. S., Coulton, C. J., Juknialis, B. W., & Leary, M. (1989). Brain death and organ retrieval: A cross-sectional survey of knowledge and concepts among health professionals. *Journal of the American Medical Association, 261,* 2205–2210.

2

COST CONTAINMENT FOR TRANSPLANT RECIPIENTS

Sara J. Munk, R.N., B.S.N.

Cost containment in transplantation is essential in order to be competitive in today's health care market. Gone are the days of unlimited benefits, long lengths of stay, and inpatient rather than outpatient focus. Most hospitals with transplant programs are re-evaluating their standards of practice and redefining the minimal, essential practice needed to provide high-quality patient outcomes.

INCENTIVES FOR CHANGE

Two common incentives for cost containment in the hospital setting are third-party payors and administrative budget reduction. A growing number of larger insurance companies are establishing centers of excellence. These centers are hospitals located nationwide that provide specialized services such as transplantation. These centers of excellence have specific criteria such as a minimum number of cases per year and quality of life indicators that confirm positive patient outcomes in transplantation. The insurance company then seeks out those facilities, providing high-quality patient outcomes with the lowest costs. The consensus is that the facilities performing the greatest number of cases are more proficient, have higher quality patient outcomes, and have lower costs due to their efficiency. Hospital administration strives to maintain a low cost per case to ensure contracts for transplantation. This will increase the number of cases performed per year and therefore positions the hospital to receive more contracts, particularly those based on centers of excellence. Bottom line—low cost and high patient quality outcomes will create more business for the hospital.

COST CONTAINMENT MEASURES

How, then, do you reduce your costs? By defining medical practice by what is essential and what is not. The most frequent and efficient ways to achieve lower costs without reducing quality of patient care are utilization review, case management, clinical pathways, and outpatient services (see Figure 2.1).

Utilization Review

Decreasing utilization can bring about tremendous decreases in costs. Early extubation; minimizing laboratory studies, chest x-rays, and electrocardiograms; and revision of antibiotic therapy all contribute to lower-

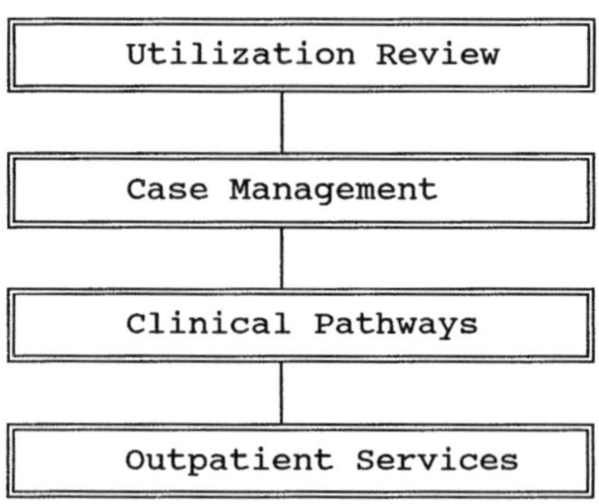

FIGURE 2.1 Cost containment measures.

ing costs. Isolation practices have been reduced significantly, allowing transplant patients to be roomed with other noninfected patients. This is especially important because it reduces hours of nursing care and, in combination with all the above listed initiatives, can decrease the length of stay in the intensive care unit, which costs approximately $2,000 per day compared to a transition/intermediate care unit costing $1,100 to 1,300 per day.

Case Management

Early implementation of case management focuses on identifying discharge needs of a patient and makes certain these arrangements are in place to streamline services and facilitate early discharge by reducing duplication. Case managers provide needed information to the patient and form links between the patient, the insurance company, and the health care network. They facilitate communication between the hospital and insurance companies by providing appropriate information such as patient condition, estimated length of stay, complications, and any discharge needs that are anticipated. This proactive strategy helps to alleviate miscommunication and diminishes anxiety for the patient, whose primary focus should be his/her health, not finance and system issues.

Clinical Pathways

Clinical pathways employ the essential practice standards identified by the health care team. (See an example from Stanford Health Services—Table 2.1.) All aspects of care, such as blood work, studies, activity, diet, medications, etc., are outlined onto a timeline. This timeline can be hourly or daily. Each category has an expected clinical outcome that needs to be attained. If the outcome is not attained, a variance occurs. These variances are tracked, and the goal is to expedite the patient back into the pathway as quickly as possible.

There are three types of variances: patient, system, and environmental. Tracking variances is very important, as it allows the staff to determine why the variance occurred and thereby evaluate if something needs to be changed on the pathway or if there are system failures that might need to be addressed. This promotes continual evaluation of patient care and allows care providers to take steps quickly to optimize patient care. The pathways incorporate a multitude of services such as physician, nurse, physical/occupational therapist, pharmacist, and dietitian. Each can easily access the pathway and, in conjunction with preprinted standing

TABLE 2.1 Clinical Pathways: Uncomplicated Heart Transplant

VARIANCE SUMMARY:
PATIENT VARIANCE ______ SYSTEM/CAREGIVER VARIANCE ______

	PRE-OP	DOS	POD 1	POD 2	POD 3	POD 4
Patient Variance: Explanation Action Plan						
System Variance: Action Plan						
Vital Signs	Q 4 hr	Q 30 min x 12 hr Q 1 hr x 12	Q 2 hr	Q 4 hr (Q 2 hr while weaning isuprel)	Q 4 hr (Q 2 hr while weaning isuprel	Q 4 hr
Ventilation		ventilator $ETCO_2$ oximetry 1 ABG-admission 1 ABG-CPAP	extubated mask 02 oximetry 1 ABG extubation inspirometer	mask O_2 or nasal cannula D/C oximetry inspirometer Q 2-4 hr w/a	mask O_2 or nasal cannula inspirometer Q 2-4 hrs w/a	D/C 02
Monitor		continuous	continuous	continuous	continuous or overview	continuous or overview
Monitoring Lines / Drains		CVP line PA line peripheral IV chest tubes foley NG tube pacing wires	CVP line PA line D/C peripheral IV D/C chest tubes D/C foley D/C NG tube pacing wires	triple lumen CVP D/C PA line pacing wires	triple lumen CVP pacing wires	triple lumen CVP pacing wire
Laboratory / Studies	labs per research protocols routine transplant medication per protocol.......› immunosuppressants until discharge					
Medications		antibiotics isuprel infusion inotrope vasodilator IV pain mgmt	antibiotics isuprel infusion wean inotrope wean vasodilator IV pain mgmt	antibiotics isupril infusion IV/PO pain mgmt	D/C antibiotics isuprel infusion PO pain mgmt until discharge	
Activity	up ad lib	bedrest	up in chair/dangle	up in chair	ambulation in rm	ambulate in hall
Diet	NPO	NPO	clear liquids advance to full liquid	advance to regular (low na, low chol)	regular	regular
Teaching				begin review of drugs with pt. & spouse give teaching booklet	begin exercise instruction	pt. begins to identify drugs by name
Placement	D2, CSU	ICU	ICU	ICU	ICU	transfer to D2
Consults				case manager	PT consult social worker dietician	pt consult

(continued)

orders, minimize delays, repetition, and unwarranted services. This is particularly helpful in academic settings with large numbers of medical students and new residents, because it helps control utilization and is used as a teaching tool to help them focus on what lab work, studies, etc., are pertinent. Clinical pathways are more readily used on uncomplicated

TABLE 2.1 *(continued)*

VARIANCE SUMMARY:
PATIENT VARIANCE ______ SYSTEM/CAREGIVER VARIANCE ______

	POD 5	POD 6	POD 7	POD 8	POD 9	POD 10	POD 11
Patient Variance: Explanation Action Plan							
System Variance: Action Plan							
Vital Signs	Q 6 hr	Q 6 hr	Q 6 hr	Q 8 hr post neg biopsy	Q 8 hr	Q 8 hr	
Ventilation	rooom air..............................›						
Monitor	telemetry..............................›						
Monitoring Lines / Drains	heparin lock to CVP pacing wires	heparin lock pacing wires	heparin lock pacing wires	heparin lock pacing wires	heparin lock pacing wires	heparin lock D/C pacing wires	D/C CVP
Laboratory / Studies			biopsy				
Medications	routine transplant medications per protocol..............................discharge medications from Pharmacy						
Activity	exercise protocol per PT..............................›						
Diet	regular nas (low fat, low chol)..............................›						
Teaching	reinforce material in transplant teaching booklet..............................self admin. of medication						
Placement	D2	D2	D2	D2	D2	D2	discharge
Consults	PT conslut	PT consult			schedule OKT3 therapy in ATU POD 12-14 dietician	appt for 2nd biopsy & coronary studies, transplant coord. pre-clinic visit	

Source: Stanford University Hospital Department of Nursing, Stanford, CA.

kidney and heart transplant patients. They become very complex with the lung, liver, kidney/pancreas, and bone marrow transplant patients because there are a multitude of variances to track with the more complicated multisystem transplantation.

Outpatient Services

Finally, the largest growth in today's health care market is the shift to an outpatient focus. Previously, patients were required to be hospitalized 2 to 4 weeks post-transplantation, receiving multiple biopsies and IV drug administration and refining their immunosuppression drug regimen. The longer they were required to remain in the hospital, the greater the chance of nosocomial infections in their immunosuppressed state. The trend is for early discharge if the patient is stable. Kidney transplant recipients are released after 4 to 5 days. Heart transplants without complications and with negative biopsies are being discharged in 8 to 9 days post-transplant. We are now able to facilitate these early discharges because of the extensive and specialized care that can be given in outpatient settings, such as ambulatory treatment units within a clinic or hospital and the home itself. Intravenous medications such as OKT3 and cytotoxins are limited to the hospital setting per federal regulation, but because they are rarely given more than twice a day, it provides the opportunity for the patient to stay in local housing and have these therapies provided in the ambulatory treatment unit. Most patients prefer this rather than staying in the hospital. Most hospitals with transplant programs have set aside local housing, an apartment, or a hotel room with convenient shuttle service. All these details are part of the transplant package allowing frequent clinic visits both pre- and post-transplantation. Those patients who are fortunate enough to live close to a transplant center often are able to use home care as an option. Insurance companies prefer this direction of outpatient services and have at times amended coverage to provide these outpatient services. The cost savings are tremendous. Compare a nursing visit charge of $125 to an inpatient day on a postsurgical floor of $800 to $1,200. This focus on outpatient services will only increase as budget reductions continue to occur and national health care becomes a reality.

SUMMARY

Cost containment initiatives in transplantation are an ongoing process. At Stanford Health Services, we have used the above methods for the last four years and have successfully decreased the length of stay for heart transplants from $24\frac{4}{10}$ days in 1990 to $17\frac{6}{10}$ days in 1993. If our outliers were removed, the length of stay decreases further to $12\frac{1}{2}$ days. (Outliers are defined as patients with length of stay greater than 20 days.) We are currently establishing clinical pathways in multi-organ and bone marrow transplants, refining our heart transplant clinical pathway and incorporating it into a computer charting system.

3

IMPROVEMENTS IN DISCHARGE PLANNING AND HOME HEALTH CARE

Pam McFarlin, R.N., M.S.N.

Caring for patients at home is the oldest form of health care. Nurses have been making home visits since about the 1890s. However, during the past 10 to 15 years, there has been a dramatic change in the kinds of care provided in the home and the number of home health agencies available to provide the care.

> Definition of Home Health Care
>
> Home Health Care is defined as "skilled nursing and other therapeutic services providing care to patients in their homes on a part-time or intermittent basis under a plan of treatment as prescribed by the attending physician." (Medicare Conditions of Participation for Home Health Care, 1989)

The goals of the home care team are for the patient to learn self-care and become as independent as possible. In many cases, this will involve one or more residential caregivers and the patient, who are taught and supported by the home care team.

HOME CARE TEAM

Skilled Caregivers

- Registered nurse
- Home health aide
- Physical therapist
- Licensed vocational nurse
- Occupational therapist
- Physician
- Speech therapist
- Volunteer
- Medical social worker

Residential Caregivers

- Spouse
- Children
- Friends
- Attendants

Services provided to patients in the home include skilled nursing, skilled therapy, home health aide, medical social worker, and volunteer services. The physician may make home visits but usually is overseeing the care through telecommunication with the home care staff.

TRAINING

The training of the skilled home care team varies according to the individual staff member's past experience and discipline. Home health aides are certified nursing assistants who have received additional training and licensure. They provide personal care and other duties at home under the supervision of the registered nurse or therapist.

Registered nurses and licensed vocational nurses represent the largest percentage of skilled caregivers in the home. Hospital-based home care programs have advantages over nonhospital programs because the nursing staff can be cross-trained to work in home care, therefore meeting the demand for highly skilled personnel. Nurses not coming from an acute setting need to have a broad background with several years of experience, preferably in home care. Other home care staff require an intensive orientation and additional training as needed. Training tends to be ongoing as care at home becomes more complex.

Residential caregivers receive on-site training from the home care staff. Caregiver classes are offered in the community through adult education and senior centers. Caregivers who have been hired through an agency will receive training through the employer and specific patient training from the home care staff.

RESPONSIBILITIES OF THE HOME CARE TEAM

During the past decade, home health care has become high-technique, high-touch. It provides the same care at home that 5 or 10 years ago was provided in an acute hospital or skilled nursing facility. Care provided includes the following:

- Wound care
- Patient assessment
- Diabetic care
- Teaching of medication
- Stoma care
- Supportive care of the dying
- Therapies: physical, occupational, and speech
- Infusion services
- Pulmonary toilet

Visits to the home may be as often as four times a day or as little as once a month. Private insurance, Medicare, and Medicaid pay for home care with little or no cost to the patient.

Although home care provides high-tech services, these are performed in a simpler, more comfortable and economical way (Rothkopf, 1992). The biggest advancement in the home health care practice has been the development of home infusion. Home infusion includes, but is not limited to, treatments such as total parenteral nutrition (TPN), antibiotics, chemotherapy, cardiac medications, and blood products.

Shorter lengths of stay and economic trends have been the indicators for the increase in home care visits. Patients or caregivers generally are receptive and do extremely well learning even the most complex home care programs. Patients, when given the choice, usually would rather be cared for at home than in the hospital. Home care is available to patients both very young and very old and can be provided 24 hours per day, 7 days per week. Home health care staff can provide information to the patient regarding community resources and attendant care in the home when needed.

HOME CARE AND THE TRANSPLANT

The development of high-tech home care has made it possible to provide care at home for transplant patients, both pre- and post-transplant. Assessment prior to admission to the transplant program includes assessing home support systems, the patient's ability to learn, and the willingness to assume self-care. Due to the long-term care needs of most transplant patients, these patients will be likely recipients of home care services.

Home Infusion

Patients, pre- or post-transplant, requiring home infusion will be evaluated for suitability by the physician, the transplant team, and the home liaison nurse. In order to qualify for home infusion, a patient must be able to learn certain aspects of the care to be considered safe. Patients unable to learn must have an available and willing residential caregiver at all times who will be taught how to troubleshoot problems. Patients receiving long-term or complex therapy need to have a permanent vascular access device in place.

Once it has been determined that the patient is suitable to receive infusion therapy at home, the drug is evaluated for stability once mixed and to assess whether or not the drug can be infused using an ambulatory pump such as a CADD, a portable infusion pump with medication cassette manufactured by Pharmacia Deltec, Inc.

CADD—Portable IV Infusion Pump

- Battery operated
- Size of Walkman radio
- Lockout safety features
- Carry in a "fanny-pack" worn around the waist

The use of the ambulatory pump is the most cost-effective. It is simple to learn to operate. The pump allows the patient to be mobile and go about normal activities of daily living. The pump can be programmed to give doses of medicine as often as needed and infusion at a minimal keep-open rate in between doses. The pump can also be programmed to run consistently when necessary to infuse hydration, TPN, or pain medication. The pump is programmed by the home infusion staff and is locked into place, making it safe to use.

Teaching a patient and/or caregiver about using the pump will depend on the patient's learning capacity and willingness to learn.

Minimum teaching includes the following:

- Troubleshooting alarms
- Turning off the pump
- Calling the home care nurse

Maximum teaching includes learning to do the following:

- Changing the cassettes on the pump
- Changing the tubing
- Rotating the site, if subcutaneous
- Mixing the medication

Teaching for these home infusions is begun while the patient is still in the hospital. The day the patient is discharged, the home care nurse visits in the evening to continue teaching and orient the patient and caregiver to the home care program. Subsequent teaching and home visits will be determined at the initial visit and a plan of care developed.

HOME CARE PROCEDURES FOR THE TRANSPLANT PATIENT

Following are examples of some procedures currently being performed successfully in the home care setting.

Pretransplant

Pulmonary Toilet for Lung Transplant Candidates. Lung transplant candidates may require daily or twice daily aggressive chest physiotherapy, which can be performed by the home care nurse. In addition, the frequent monitoring by the staff in the home may identify problems and ensure immediate follow-up.

Dobutamine for Heart Transplant Candidates. Some candidates, due to poorly functioning hearts, may need continuous intravenous infusion of dobutamine to keep them out of cardiac failure (Phillips, 1992).

Patients who are stable enough may remain at home on a continuous dobutamine infusion via an ambulatory pump. This can be achieved either by self-administration or with the assistance of a caregiver.

Post-transplant

Ganciclovir for Cytomegalovirus Infections. Cytomegalovirus (CMV) infection is common in immunocompromised patients and is treated by giving patients ganciclovir (DHPG) intravenously. This drug is most commonly given by gravity infusion, and the patient or caregiver is taught to infuse.

TPN for Nutritional Depletion. The post-transplant patient who is stable enough to leave the hospital, but who still requires nutritional or hydration support, is able to do so with the services provided by the home care team.

FUTURE TRENDS IN HOME CARE AND THE TRANSPLANT PATIENT

An example of future trends is autologous stem cell infusions for the treatment of advanced breast cancer. Until recently, this was done as a totally inpatient procedure. It is now being done at some hospitals as an outpatient procedure due to the support of high-tech home care.

Patients come into the ambulatory treatment center to receive blood products if needed, to be evaluated for complications, and to have the high-dose chemotherapy bags changed. In the evening, the home care nurse makes a visit to evaluate the patient, draw labs, and change the hydration bag. The home care nurse is available 24 hours a day if problems or questions arise. The success of protocols such as this one is dependent on a dedicated team, including the patient and the home care staff.

COLLABORATIVE CARE IN THE OUTPATIENT SETTING

Some hospitals and clinics have ambulatory treatment or infusion centers where mobile patients can go to receive infusion therapy. When it is possible for the medication to be infused via an ambulatory pump, it is more desirable for the patient to remain at home and receive care. When a patient is receiving multiple therapies, including blood transfusions and several-hour drip infusions, the patient will go to the center in the morning and receive home care for the evening dose of medication. Some insurance companies are willing to pay for both treatments because the cost is still less expensive and more desirable than hospitalization.

SUMMARY

The future of home health care has no boundaries. Integrated information systems linking the patient, the physician, and the home care agency will enable the same continuity to prevail as in the hospital setting at a lower cost and in a more desirable setting. Home care agencies act as resources for locating special-duty workers who can provide up to 24-hour care in the home and for coordinating all the care needed. As the health care dollar becomes smaller and outpatient services become more sophisticated, patients will be able to receive the highest level of care while remaining at home.

REFERENCES

Federal Registrar. Department of Health & Human Services, Healthcare Financing Administration. (1989). *Medicare Conditions of Participation for Home Health Care.* Washington, DC.

Phillips, P. (1992). Home dobutamine. *Canadian Nurse,* 13–5.

Rothkopf, M. M. (1992). Intensive home care. *New Jersey Medicine,* 31–34.

4

LONG-TERM RECOVERY ISSUES FOLLOWING TRANSPLANTATION

D. Kathryn Tierney, R.N., M.S.N.

Organ transplantation has become a widely employed technology for a variety of end-stage organ failure states and certain malignant and non-malignant disorders of the lymphohematopoietic system. Long-term health consequences facing individuals undergoing transplant need to be clearly understood now if recovery issues are to be minimized in the future. This chapter will describe what is known about the long-term health consequences of bone marrow and solid organ transplantation and identify areas needing further investigation.

Over 35,000 individuals have received allogeneic bone marrow transplants since the mid-1950s, and the number increases steadily (Bortin, Horowitz, & Rimm, 1992). The use of bone marrow transplant as a therapeutic option began in the 1970s and rapidly grew during the 1980s as our knowledge of histocompatibility typing, supportive care, and immunosuppressive therapy expanded. Similarly, the use of organ transplantation for a variety of end-stage organ diseases grew with improvements in surgical techniques, antibiotic and immunosuppressive therapy, and organ procurement and preservation. In 1993, the United Network for Organ Sharing reported that 18,164 solid organ transplants were performed. Kidney transplants accounted for 10,928 (60%), liver transplants 3,442 (19%), pancreas transplants 772 (4%), heart grafts 2,298 (13%), heart-lung transplants 60 (<1%) and lung transplants 664 (3%) (Slack, 1994).

Success in bone marrow transplant (BMT) is dependent on a number of variables, including recipient disease status and overall state of health. Allogeneic BMT for hematologic malignancies is more successful if carried out while the patient is in complete remission for acute leukemia or in the chronic phase of chronic myelogenous leukemia. Sixty-five percent of patients with acute leukemia transplanted in first complete remission will obtain a cure, and 70% of patients receiving a matched sibling transplant for chronic myelogenous leukemia in first chronic phase will be cured. Land reports that 80 to 90% of cadaver kidney transplants survive 1 year, with a 6-year graft survival rate of 51% (Land, 1989). A 2-year survival rate of 60 to 70% is reported following single- or double-lung transplants and heart-lung transplants (Williams, Grossman, & Maurer, 1990). One-year survival for liver transplant patients is reported at 83% and 5-year survival ranges from 65 to 71% (Knechtle et al., 1993). Seventy-eight percent of cardiac transplant recipients survive 1 year, and 73% survive 5 years (Muirhead, 1989).

The immunosuppressive therapies employed in the field of transplantation will be reviewed. This review will cover the infectious risks and the risk of cancer development as a result of ongoing immunosuppressive therapy. Chronic graft rejection following solid organ transplants and chronic graft-versus-host disease following BMT will be reviewed in detail because they remain a major source of morbidity and mortality following transplantation. Focus will then shift to other health problems experienced during recovery following transplantation; and finally, return to work, sexual satisfaction, and quality of life issues will be addressed.

The above list of long-term health risks highlights the vital role nurses have to play in the informed consent process. Long before aggressive pretransplant workups are initiated, the patient and family must be given a detailed explanation of the entire process. Short- and long-term effects must be explained, and nurses must develop some means of assessing the patients' and families' understanding. Informed consent does not happen in a single visit or interview, but continues slowly and steadily throughout the pretransplant phase.

IMMUNOSUPPRESSIVE THERAPY

There is a wide variety of immunosuppressive agents available for clinical use and many more are in various stages of development. As newer and more precise agents become available, many of the issues now faced by transplant recipients will become part of the history of transplantation. Agents that specifically target those components of the immune system responsible for graft-versus-host disease (GVHD) or graft rejection, and spare other components of the immune system responsible for removal of infectious organisms and tumor surveillance, will be a major breakthrough in the field of transplantation. While these speculations on the future of immunosuppressive therapy are exciting, a review of the current therapy is valuable if, as nurses, we are to help prepare our patients not only for the immediate post-transplant period, but for their recovery as well.

Cyclosporine A

Cyclosporine A (CsA) is a potent immunosuppressive agent that profoundly affects cellular immunity. It specifically decreases the number of cytotoxic T cells and inhibits the function of helper T cells. Interleukin-1 and interleukin-2 production and release are blocked by CsA (Pillon, 1991). It is nephrotoxic, and monitoring of the creatinine and blood urea nitrogen is essential to avoid irreversible kidney damage. The nurse needs to make a frequent review of the patient's medication profile and monitor the use of the additional nephrotoxic drugs. Other signs of nephrotoxicity include hyperkalemia, fluid retention, prolonged creatinine clearance, hematuria, and acidosis (Pillon, 1991). Hypertension will be observed in almost all patients, especially when the medication is initiated and doses are generally higher. Antihypertensive therapy will be essential, and the nurse should review the rationale for therapy as well as expected signs and symptoms with the patient. Hepatic toxicity is demonstrated by increases in serum bilirubin, alkaline phosphatase, and transaminases. Hepatic toxicity is generally reversible with adjustments in the CsA dose. Seizures are a rare complication of CsA therapy; but tremors, particularly of the hands, are common. Hyperpigmentation and increased facial hair growth are side effects of CsA that can have negative effects on the patient's body image and self-esteem. Headaches and gingival hyperplasia may be noted (Sheets, 1989). Gastrointestinal disturbances include nausea, vomiting, anorexia, and an unpleasant taste. These generally subside as the dosage is decreased toward maintenance levels. In addition, a tablet form of CsA is now available that is not associated with the unpleasant taste of the liquid suspension. Maintenance doses range from 5 to 10 mg/kg/day, but are variable depending upon the treating physician's practice and patient tolerance.

Corticosteroids

Corticosteroids are immunosuppressive agents used in the prevention and treatment of both acute and chronic graft rejection and GVHD. Effects of corticosteroids on the immune system are diverse. Both cellular and humoral immunity are affected, and the inflammatory response is depressed. Prednisone inhibits interleukin-1 production and antigen presentation (Sheets, 1989). Neutrophil chemotaxis is also impaired with the use of corticosteroids. Side effects are reviewed in Table 4.1. Helping patients comply with a medication regimen with such a long list of side effects is challenging. Patients with a good understanding of the benefits of maintaining their immunosuppressive therapy will be better able to cope with the side effects. Adolescents and young adults are at particular risk for difficulty coping with the changes in body image, and nurses must direct their efforts in helping to assure compliance with therapy and encouraging positive coping strategies. Advising patients to take the prednisone with antacids, milk, or food will decrease the risk of peptic ulcer formation. Sleep disturbances and mood swings are most problematic during the initiation of corticosteroid therapy and generally decrease when maintenance doses are reached.

Azathioprine

Azathioprine is infrequently used in BMT but is used often in solid organ transplant. Its primary use in solid organ transplants is during phases of acute rejection and maintenance therapy. Azathioprine inhibits cellular immunity by decreasing the function of activated T cells. The most significant side effect is bone marrow suppression. Dosage adjustments are

TABLE 4.1 Long-Term Side Effects of Corticosteroids

• Impaired wound healing	• Muscle atrophy
• Cataracts	• Osteoporosis
• Fluid and sodium retention	• Mood swings
• Hypertension	• Sleep disturbances
• Peptic ulcer disease	• Body image disturbances
• Diabetes mellitus	• Acne
• Aseptic necrosis of joints	• Hyperlipidemia

made based on the individual's white blood cell count. Other side effects include liver abnormalities and alopecia (Harasyko, 1989).

Most solid organ transplant patients are treated with a three-drug regimen to prevent graft rejection. This three-drug combination consists of cyclosporine A, steroids, and azathioprine (Harasyko, 1989). Prospective randomized trials need to be initiated and completed to determine the immunosuppressive therapy that results in the lowest rate of acute and chronic rejection, decreased risk of infection, minimal side effects, and a low incidence of malignancies. In BMT, GVHD prevention varies among different centers but generally includes some combination of CsA, prednisone, and methotrexate. Methotrexate is a chemotherapy agent that suppresses the growth of new T lymphocytes (Wujcik, Ballard, & Camp-Sorrell, 1994). It is administered intravenously during the first month post-BMT and is used for the prevention of acute GVHD. Unlike solid organ transplants, for those patients who have no signs or symptoms of acute or chronic GVHD, all immunosuppressive therapy will be discontinued. Tolerance between the host and graft develops in the majority of BMT patients, and immunosuppressive therapy is withdrawn at 6 months to 2 years post-transplant.

Education of the patient is a key nursing responsibility. Assuring that the patient understands not only the advantages of maintaining the immunosuppressive therapy but the risks of discontinuing therapy is of paramount importance in assuring long-term compliance. In addition to educating patients about the rationale for the medications, the nurse needs to teach them about side effects and strategies to minimize these problems. Chronic use of immunosuppressive agents leaves the host vulnerable to infectious complications because of their diverse and extensive effects on host immunity. Education of the client regarding the nature of infections, risk factors, signs and symptoms of infection, and necessary therapy is a nursing responsibility in caring for transplant recipients.

INFECTIONS

Infections remain a major source of morbidity and mortality following all types of transplantation. The high dose chemotherapy with or without radiation therapy employed in BMT to eradicate the malignancy causes an immunodeficiency that lasts for 3 to 5 months (Deeg, 1992). Full recovery of the immune system takes 2 years (Lum, 1990). Compounding the immunocompromise from the conditioning regimen is the immunosuppressive therapy employed in the prevention of GVHD. In BMT patients suffering from chronic GVHD, infectious complications are more common and carry a higher mortality. Likewise, solid organ transplant patients are vulnerable to infectious complications because of the defects in host defenses related to their immunosuppressive therapy and underlying medical conditions, such as diabetes mellitus.

For BMT and solid organ transplant recipients, infections seen from 2 to 6 months following transplant include herpes virus infections and opportunistic infections. Opportunistic pathogens including *Nocardia asteroides, Aspergillus, Listeria monocytogenes,* and *Pneumocystis carinii* (Rubin, 1993). After 6 months, infectious complications decrease in frequency because the individual is usually on low-maintenance doses of immunosuppressive therapy. The exception to this general rule is in individuals with poor graft function (Rubin, 1993) or BMT recipients with chronic GVHD, where chronic viral infections and opportunistic infections continue to present significant problems. Treatment for infections in the post-transplant period depends upon the severity of the infection and the organism involved. Generally speaking, immunosuppressed individuals need aggressive and immediate therapy to avoid rapid dissemination of infection, and antimicrobial therapy is usually prolonged beyond the resolution of the infectious episode because of the underlying immunosuppression. Rehospitalization for the treatment of infections can be physically and emotionally difficult for transplant patients who have already undergone multiple procedures, tests, and prolonged hospitalizations.

Bacterial

The respiratory system is a frequent target of bacterial infections in the BMT patient. There appears to be a relationship between infection and post-transplant lung disease, although the nature of the relationship is unclear (Krowka, Rosenow, & Hoagland, 1985; Kurzrock et al., 1984). Organisms frequently encountered include *Streptococcus pneumoniae, Haemophilus influenzae,* and *Staphylococcus aureus* (Atkinson, et al., 1979; Winston, Ho, Champlin, & Gale, 1984). Astute observation, education of the individual to seek medical assistance promptly for any symptoms of respiratory infection, judicious use of broad spectrum antibiotic therapy, and administration of intravenous immunoglobulin (Sullivan et al., 1990) help decrease the incidence of bacterial infections. Bacterial pneumonia in solid organ recipients may be observed in relationship to a period of increased immunosuppression related to the treatment of an episode of acute rejection (Dunn, 1990).

Urinary tract infections (UTI), common during the immediate postoperative period, decrease in frequency by 6 months following kidney transplant. Most UTIs require a course of oral antibiotics that can be administered on an outpatient basis (Dunn, 1990). A kidney transplant patient with a history of recurrent UTIs may benefit from a prophylactic schedule of antibiotic therapy. Treatment of *Salmonella* gastroenteritis with fluoroquinolones should be aggressively pursued in the immunocompromised individual because of its propensity to disseminate in this population (Rubin, 1993). *Listeria monocytogenes* can be a significant pathogen in individuals receiving corticosteroid therapy but can be prevented with the use of prophylactic trimethoprim-sulfamethoxazole (Rubin, 1993).

Viral

Viral infections, particularly the *varicella zoster* virus (VZV), are a major cause of morbidity in transplant patients. In BMT recipients, the disease may be localized or disseminated. Individuals experience itching, paresthesia, pain, and fever and develop a red, blistering rash that follows a dermatome. Early and prompt treatment with intravenous acyclovir helps to control the spread and minimize the disease's sequelae (Arvin, 1993). The median onset of infection is 5 months (Wingard, 1993) and occurs in up to 50% of individuals following BMT (Arvin, 1993). Complications from VZV infection include visceral or pulmonary dissemination, cranial nerve involvement, and postherpetic neuralgia. Studies are currently under way to determine the role of VZV vaccination of the BMT donor, the recipient, or both in decreasing the incidence of herpes zoster infection post-transplant (Blume & Chao, 1992). VZV infections do not differ significantly in course, presentation, or treatment in recipients of solid organ transplants.

Cytomegalovirus (CMV) infections are common in the first few months following transplant. The incidence of significant CMV disease is reported to be 10 to 30% in solid organ transplant recipients (Dunn, 1990). The incidence in BMT ranges from 66% in CMV seropositive recipients to 31% in CMV seronegative recipients, with a mortality rate as high as 50% (Quan & Bowden, 1993). Diagnosis is based on a fourfold or greater increase in CMV antibody titer, isolation of CMV for any site, or the presence of CMV inclusion bodies on tissue biopsy. Infection can occur as a result of reactivation, superinfection, or primary infection. The prognosis is least favorable for primary infection and most favorable with reactivation of the virus. Prophylactic administration of CMV immunoglobulin for the first several months following transplant has decreased the incidence of CMV disease in kidney transplant recipients (Snydman et al., 1987). Other prophylactic measures include using a CMV-negative donor; this may be more of an option in BMT than solid organ transplant and the use of CMV-negative blood products. Presenting symptoms may be mild and include fever, leukopenia, malaise, and myalgia, or be more severe with interstitial pneumonitis, pneumonia, pancreatitis, hepatitis, and retinitis (Dunn, 1990; Quan & Bowden, 1993). Gastroduodenal ulcers may develop in the upper or lower gastrointestinal (GI) tract as a result of CMV infection resulting in perforation and bleeding (Dunn, 1990). Approximately 12% of BMT recipients will develop CMV infection of the GI tract (Quan & Bowden, 1993). The esophagus is most frequently involved, characterized by persistent nausea and vomiting. Ganciclovir and immunoglobulin preparations are used in the treatment of CMV infection. Foscarnet is another medication that can be used. Nursing care, support, and education are important during this treatment course, which may extend up to 3 months. Daily visits to the ambulatory treatment center are required for the administration of these intravenous medications. A second option may be to instruct the patient on self-administration for home infusion therapy. Bone marrow suppression may follow the administration of ganciclovir, and monitoring the complete blood count is necessary.

In addition to the problems viral infections cause in and of themselves in transplant recipients, viral infections may predispose BMT recipients to GVHD (Atkinson, 1992) and appear to increase the rate of graft rejection in heart transplants (Grattan et al., 1989). A role for viruses in the development of malignancies in the immunocompromised host is also under investigation. A strong association between primary or reactivation of Epstein-Barr virus infections and the development of lymphoproliferative malignancies has been described (Starzl et al., 1984).

Protozoan and Parasitic Pathogens

The use of prophylactic trimethoprim-sulfamethoxazole or inhaled pentamidine has significantly reduced the incidence of pneumonitis caused by the *Pneumocystis carinii* organism in immunocompromised hosts.

Fungal

Fungal infections following transplant are common and range in severity from mild to life-threatening. Organisms seen include *Candida* species, *Aspergillus* species, *Cryptococcus, Histoplasma,* and *Nocardia.* Sites of fungal infection include the oral cavity, esophagus, blood, sinuses, lungs, and central nervous system. The use of immunosuppressive medication for the prevention and treatment of GVHD and chronic rejection, and broad-spectrum antibiotic use, contribute to the risk of fungal infections and make treatment more difficult.

Candidal infections are common in the immunocompromised transplant recipient and frequently involve the oral cavity. Prophylactic administration of an oral antifungal agent may avoid this problem and should be administered during periods of increased immunosuppression or during therapy for a bacterial infection (Dunn, 1990). *Candida* may also infect the urinary tract, and topical amphotericin B therapy is warranted. If symptoms persist, systemic therapy may be indicated (Dunn, 1990).

Aspergillus pneumonia is a life-threatening event. The reported incidence is 18 to 55% with a mortality of 80% (Krowka, Rosenow, & Hoagland, 1985). The portal of entry is the respiratory tract, but in the immunocompromised host, the disease can rapidly disseminate to the blood or central nervous system (CNS). Amphotericin B is the treatment of choice. Whether to reduce or discontinue the immunosuppressive medications is a difficult clinical choice because the risks of losing the graft or the development of GVHD are serious consequences requiring consideration. Treatment of fungal infections usually requires a prolonged course of therapy. Antifungal agents include amphotericin B, 5-Fluorocytosine, ketoconazole, fluconazole, and itraconazole. It should be remembered that ketoconazole and itraconazole will increase CsA levels, and close monitoring is essential.

Infectious complications following transplant represent a major therapeutic challenge. Nurses play a role in patient education, administration of antimicrobial therapy, minimizing and monitoring the side effects of therapy, preventing complications, and providing emotional support.

CHRONIC GRAFT-VERSUS-HOST DISEASE

Chronic graft-versus-host disease [GVHD] is a systemic multiorgan disorder that affects 20 to 50% (Atkinson, 1992; Chao, 1992) of individuals following HLA-identical sibling BMT. Clinically, chronic GVHD can range from a limited and mild disorder to an extensive, severe, and fatal condition. Half of those individuals with chronic GVHD have minimal involvement, while 15% have severe disease (Atkinson et al., 1990).

Pathophysiology

The pathophysiology of chronic GVHD is the result of a dynamic and complex interaction between the host and donor graft. Chronic GVHD shares many clinical similarities to a variety of autoimmune and collagen vascular disorders. Clinically, the disorder has features of systemic lupus erythematosus, sicca syndrome, rheumatoid arthritis, and primary biliary sclerosis (Sullivan, 1986). GVHD is initiated by T lymphocytes recognizing and reacting to histocompatible differences on the host's tissue. Chronic GVHD causes a multifactorial immunodeficiency (see Table 4.2). On biopsy of involved tissue, three histological features noted are epithelial damage, infiltration by mononuclear cells, and fibrosis (Atkinson, 1990). The profound immunodeficiency that results from chronic GVHD and the immunosuppressive therapy used to control and treat the disease leave the host extremely vulnerable to infection. Infection remains the major cause of morbidity and mortality in individuals with chronic GVHD.

Grading

Chronic GVHD may develop at any time during the first year following allogeneic BMT. By classic definition, acute GVHD occurs within the first 100 days following marrow infusion, and chronic GVHD develops after 100 days. Clinically, however, chronic GVHD has been observed as early as 40 days (Ferrara & Deeg, 1991) and as late as 15 months after transplant (Atkinson, 1990). The median onset is 3 to 4 months after marrow transplantation. The grading scale for chronic GVHD is divided into two categories: those with limited disease and those with extensive disease. Limited disease is confined to the skin with or without liver involvement.

TABLE 4.2 Characteristics of the Immunodeficiency of Chronic Graft-Versus-Host Disease

- Decreased number of T lymphocytes
- Decreased function of T lymphocytes
- Decreased production of immunoglobulin
- Impaired thymic function
- Increased nonspecific suppressor cell activity
- Impaired chemotaxis of neutrophils
- Impaired antibody production
- Presence of alloreactive T cells
- Presence of autoreactive T cells
- Development of autoantibodies

Source: Adapted and modified from: "Graft-Versus-Host Disease," by J. L. M. Ferrara and H. J. Deeg, 1991, *The New England Journal of Medicine, 324. Graft-Versus-Host Disease*, by N. J. Chao, 1994, Austin: R. G. Landes Company. "Chronic Graft-Versus-Host Disease," by K. Atkinson, 1990, *Bone Marrow Transplantation, 5.*

Disease that includes other organ systems is defined as extensive. Limited chronic GVHD is associated with a favorable outcome, and the value of treatment in limited disease is debated (Atkinson, 1990; Chao, 1992). Extensive chronic GVHD is associated with a poor prognosis, with a mortality rate from progression of the disease and associated infections approaching 75% (Chao, 1992).

Risk Factors

Risk factors and prognostic indicators for chronic GVHD have been defined. Risk factors for the development of chronic GVHD include all risk factors associated with acute GVHD (see Table 4.3), older recipient age, infusion of donor buffy coat, CMV infection, infusion of CMV positive marrow, and prior acute GVHD. A strong correlation between acute GVHD and the development of the chronic form exists. The incidence of chronic GVHD in individuals with no prior acute GVHD is approximately 30% and increases to 85% in individuals with severe acute GVHD (Atkinson et al., 1990). Three patterns of association have been defined. Progressive chronic GVHD indicates that the acute disease progresses to a chronic form without interruption. Progressive GVHD is associated with an unfavorable outcome (Ferrara & Deeg, 1991; Vogelsang & Wagner, 1990; Wingard et al., 1989). Chronic GVHD that occurs after resolution of an acute episode is referred to as quiescent, and de novo chronic GVHD occurs without any prior acute GVHD (Atkinson, 1992; Vogelsang & Wagner, 1990). Other prognostic features associated with an unfavorable outcome include lichenoid skin changes, persistent severe thrombocytopenia, failure to respond to treatment, an elevated serum bilirubin, and extensive disease (Wingard et al., 1989).

Clinical Manifestations

The clinical manifestations of chronic GVHD involve the skin, liver, mouth, eyes, lungs, GI tract, neuromuscular system, vagina, kidneys and bladder, and the hematopoietic system. The organs most commonly affected are the skin and liver. There are two forms of integumentary involvement based on histology and presentation. The first is a sclerodermatous reaction. Individuals have collagen deposits with the loss of dermal appendages and atrophy. Clinically, these individuals present with loss of sweat, patchy alopecia, areas of hyperpigmentation or hypopigmentation, and thickened skin. Individuals with lichenoid skin changes of chronic GVHD present with raised papules and diffuse or patchy

TABLE 4.3 Risk Factors for Acute Graft-Versus-Host Disease

- HLA Disparity
- Opposite Gender Donor
- Age > 30 Years

erythema. On biopsy, the specimen demonstrates bandlike infiltrates of lymphocytes into the dermis. This form may progress to the sclerodermatous type reaction (Vogelsang & Wagner, 1990). In advanced cases of skin involvement, the fibrosis that is characteristic of chronic GVHD can result in joint contracture, skin ulcerations, and delayed wound healing (Atkinson, 1992). Sunlight may trigger the development of chronic skin GVHD, and therefore nurses must advise patients to use a sunscreen with a protective factor of at least 15 and protective clothing for at least the first year following BMT. The goal of nursing care for the individual with chronic skin GVHD is to maintain the integrity of the integument and prevent infection. Counseling patients to inspect the skin frequently, use mild soaps, perform range of motion exercises, and protect the skin from injury are key elements in maintaining the skin integrity and minimizing infections.

Hepatic involvement occurs frequently in individuals with chronic GVHD. A biopsy of involved tissue reveals a pattern consistent with primary biliary sclerosis and hepatitis. Laboratory values will reflect increases in the serum bilirubin and alkaline phosphatase. Liver involvement is usually limited and the disease rarely progresses to cirrhosis (Atkinson, 1990).

Involvement of the oral mucosa and salivary glands is also common. On inspection, the oral cavity may show leukoplakia, erythema, mucosal atrophy, and painful ulceration. Decreased salivary flow as a result of the destruction of the salivary glands leaves individuals with a dry mouth and a sensitivity to hot or spicy foods. Nurses need to monitor the nutritional status of the individual carefully, counsel the individual on diet modifications, and refer the patient to a nutrition therapist as appropriate. The individual should be instructed on using an oral care regimen to provide moisture and minimize discomfort. Decreased salivary flow leaves individuals more prone to dental caries, and therefore more frequent dental exams will be required. There is a delicate balance of factors in the individual with chronic GVHD between immunosuppression, malnutrition, and infection; and the nurse needs to take a proactive role in preventing and minimizing complications.

Ocular involvement results in decreased tear formation. Individuals complain of dryness and a gritty feeling. The most frequently observed ocular complication is keratoconjunctivitis sicca (Atkinson, 1992). The

Schirmer's test can be used to monitor tear production and should be administered frequently for evidence of disease progression. Nurses should instruct patients on the use of artificial tears to maintain moisture to the conjunctiva and glasses to shield the eyes from dust and foreign debris. The sicca syndrome seen in chronic GVHD often extends to the sinuses. This dryness predisposes the individual to infections, especially gram-positive bacteria. Repeated episodes of sinusitis require the use of prophylactic antibiotics, and surgical drainage may be necessary (Atkinson, 1992). Neuromuscular involvement by chronic GVHD is rare. Case reports of polymyositis, myasthenia gravis, and peripheral neuropathy have appeared in the literature (Anderson et al., 1982; Bolger et al., 1986; Greenspan et al., 1990). Other rare manifestations reported are nephrotic syndrome and severe cystitis (Gomez-Garcia et al., 1988; Ruutu, Ruutu, Volin, & Leskinen, 1988). In children and adolescents, chronic GVHD causes delays in growth and development and endocrine dysfunction. The lymphohematopoietic system may be involved as well. Laboratory data reveal eosinophilia and thrombocytopenia. The destruction of the lymphoid system can be severe. Lymphoid hypocellularity, atrophy, and a functional asplenia are seen (Atkinson, 1992). For this reason, individuals with chronic GVHD of the lymphoid system are at risk for infections with encapsulated organisms, especially pneumococcal infections.

Bronchiolitis obliterans is a rare but usually fatal complication of chronic GVHD involving the small airways of the lungs. This disorder affects approximately 10% of recipients (Holland, Wingard, Beschorner, Saral, & Santos, 1988). The patient presents with progressive dyspnea and a nonproductive cough that may quickly deteriorate to respiratory failure. Pulmonary function tests reveal a restrictive disease pattern (Atkinson, 1992). The patient's history may reveal a preceding lung infection. Holland and others found a statistically significant correlation between low serum IgG levels and the development of bronchiolitis obliterans (Holland et al., 1988). A role for prophylactic administration of intravenous immunoglobulin may be discovered through further studies (Chao, 1994). Bronchiolitis obliterans does not usually respond to immunosuppressive therapy (Atkinson, 1992).

The mucosal surfaces of the vagina may also be affected by the sicca syndrome seen with chronic GVHD. Inflammation, dryness, stricture formation, and stenosis are observed (Atkinson, 1992). Increasing the immunosuppressive therapy, dilatation, topical estrogen cream, and estrogen replacement therapy may be beneficial. Nurses can take an active role in providing the woman an opportunity to discuss any problems that exist and offer alternatives for vaginal lubrication. Involving the woman's partner in the discussions may help in allaying the fears the partner may have as well as helping both gain an understanding of the problem. A referral to a gynecologist for evaluation is warranted for any signs or symptoms of chronic GVHD of the vaginal mucosa.

The gastrointestinal (GI) tract may be affected, but is much less frequently involved than the GI involvement of acute GVHD. The individual may present with complaints of difficulty swallowing and heartburn. On x-ray, the upper esophagus is narrowed with a ring-like constriction. On tissue biopsy, the epithelial destruction characteristic of chronic GVHD of other organs is again noted (McDonald, Shulman, Sullivan, & Spencer, 1986). The lower GI tract is rarely involved except in advanced cases where symptoms include diarrhea and abdominal pain. In severe cases, malabsorption may be noted (Atkinson, 1992). Evaluating the nutritional status of the patient and his/her ability to tolerate foods and fluid, providing information on dietary modifications, and referring the individual as necessary to a nutrition counselor are all components of the nursing care plan for the individual with GI tract involvement.

Treatment

There is no consensus among bone marrow transplant physicians regarding the prevention and treatment of chronic GVHD. All rely on some combination of immunosuppressive therapy for the prevention and treatment of the disorder. Preventing the development of acute GVHD is key to preventing the chronic form. Most centers use some combination of CsA, methotrexate, prednisone, antithymocyte globulin (ATG), and T cell depletion of the marrow graft. T cell depletion is associated with a significant decrease in the incidence of acute GVHD, but its benefit is negated by a higher risk of graft rejection and relapse of disease. Current efforts are investigating the selective removal of specific subsets of T cells in the prevention of GVHD.

Treatment of established chronic GVHD involves reinstating or increasing the immunosuppressive medications. Prednisone at 2 mg/kg/day is administered for a flare-up of GVHD, and once controlled, a taper is initiated. Cyclosporine doses are adjusted as the renal and hepatic functions of the individual allow. Thalidomide has emerged as a medication with some promise in the treatment of chronic GVHD (Vogelsang et al., 1992). There have been a few positive reports on the use of ultraviolet phototherapy in the treatment of skin and oral chronic GVHD (Atkinson, Weller, Ryman, & Biggs, 1986). Other approaches include adding a cytotoxic agent such as cyclophosphamide, ATG, electron beam therapy, azathioprine, and thymic implants. Surgical approaches to the treatment of chronic

GVHD are rare, although reports exist of skin grafts and liver and lung transplantation (Griffith et al., 1993; Knobler et al., 1985; Rhodes et al., 1990).

Although chronic GVHD can be a debilitating disorder, most patients who develop chronic GVHD have limited disease and carry out their usual roles and responsibilities. There is also a benefit to GVHD in that relapse rates are noted to be lowest in individuals who have some acute and chronic graft-versus-host disease (Horowitz et al., 1990). Although the mechanism of action is not yet fully understood, it is postulated that the T cells that recognize the host as foreign will also recognize any residual leukemic cells as foreign and eliminate them. It is becoming increasingly clear that the graft-versus-leukemia (GVL) effect is an important component of the cure rates observed in allogeneic BMT. In the future, it is hoped that the GVL effect can be separated from GVHD so that cures are obtained without the problems associated with GVHD.

CHRONIC REJECTION

As in BMT, control of early or acute rejection episodes has markedly improved with the use of CsA; however, despite this development, chronic rejection constitutes a major cause of graft failure. Chronic rejection is known by many names depending upon the organ transplanted. Vanishing bile duct syndrome is the name associated with chronic rejection in liver transplant recipients. Bronchiolitis obliterans describes chronic rejection in lung transplant patients, and transplant arteriosclerosis is the name for chronic rejection of heart grafts. Chronic rejection is a progressive, uncontrollable, and irreversible immunological attack by the host that occurs despite ongoing immunosuppressive therapy (Tilney, Whitley, Diamond, Kupiec-Weglinski, & Adams, 1991). Multicenter data from Europe and the United States state that more than 50% of cadaver-derived renal transplants survived 6 years post-transplant (Land, 1989). Similarly, up to 50% of heart grafts develop coronary arteriosclerosis at 5 years (Gao et al., 1989). The incidence of chronic rejection of liver grafts appears lower, accounting for less than 10% of graft failures (Grond, Gouw, Poppema, Slooff, & Gips, 1986; Ludwig, Wiesner, Batts, Perkins, & Krom, 1987). Eight percent of single-lung transplants and 12% of double-lung grafts develop chronic rejection (Williams et al., 1990). Despite the obvious significance of chronic rejection, it is not well understood.

There is more speculation than fact on risk factors in the development of chronic rejection. In heart transplants, the ages of the donor and recipient have been suggested. HLA disparity has been implicated and supported by the observation that the rate of chronic rejection is less in kidney transplants from living donors as opposed to cadaveric donors. In a study by Kerman and others of heart transplant recipients, HLA matching did not significantly impact graft survival (Kerman et al., 1994). Hyperlipidemia, hypercholesterolemia, and high serum triglyceride levels have been studied for their roles with little conclusive evidence available to confirm or deny the association. Both CsA and corticosteroids have been implicated in the development of chronic rejection, but, again, no evidence is available to support a conclusion. The incidence of acute rejection episodes in heart transplants may be a risk factor (Gao, Schroeder, Hunt, & Stinson, 1988). The role of infection with herpes virus, particularly CMV in the early engraftment period, has been studied; and a higher rate of atherosclerosis is reported in heart transplants for those with an early CMV infection (Grattan et al., 1989).

The underlying pathology of chronic rejection is similar in kidney, heart, liver, and lung transplants. There is a progressive development of a fibrosis that obliterates the arterial vessels, which decreases blood flow to the graft (Adams & Tilney, 1989). The resulting ischemia leads to fibrotic changes within the organ and eventual failure. Coronary artery arteriosclerosis is a manifestation of a relentless immunologic attack by the host. The vessels involved develop deposits of T cells, macrophages, B cells, and smooth-muscle cells (Hruban et al., 1990). These lesions are concentric and often extend the entire length of the vessel lumen (Tilney et al., 1991). In advanced stages the myocardium shows fibrotic changes. Ultimately, recipients develop congestive heart failure, myocardial infarction, and sudden death as a result of end stage coronary artery disease (Gao et al., 1988). Recipients will not experience angina because the transplanted heart is denervated, and therefore early warning signs of coronary artery disease may not be present (Muirhead, 1989). Serial myocardial biopsies or coronary arteriograms are recommended to assess for chronic rejection.

Chronic rejection of a kidney graft may occur months to years following transplant and is manifested by gradual deterioration of kidney function, proteinuria, and hypertension (Harasyko, 1989). The process begins in the capillary lumina, which eventually narrow as a result of damage to the vascular endothelium. Fibrotic changes in the kidney occur later in the process due to ischemia (Tilney et al., 1991). Although the incidence of chronic rejection is less in liver grafts, when seen, the process is strikingly similar to what is observed in other solid organ grafts. Chronic rejection of the liver may begin months or years following transplant, and the individual may live for years without symptoms before complete graft failure or retransplantation is required (Sheets, 1989). Clinically, increasing serum bilirubin and alkaline phosphatase are noted (Grond et al., 1986). Biopsy of involved tissue reveals destructive cholangitis and the absence of bile ducts in the portal tracts (Ludwig et al., 1987). Arteriosclerotic changes are noted and extend to the larger branches of the hepatic artery. Bronchiolitis obliterans is the syndrome described in chronic rejection of lung transplants. Macrophages and lymphocytes infiltrate the bronchial lumen, resulting in fibrosis, which eventually obliterates the lumen. Both arteries and veins may be affected by arteriosclerotic changes (Tilney et al., 1991). Increasing shortness of breath, cough, and decreased exercise tolerance are noted. The pathophysiology of chronic rejection is only beginning to be described and studied. The roles of MHC antigens, mediators, humoral immunity, and adhesion molecules are unclear. As the picture that explains the pathophysiology of chronic rejection is completed, a path for therapeutic intervention will be paved.

DELAYED EFFECTS OF BONE MARROW TRANSPLANT

Many of the long-term health consequences following BMT reflect a series of insults that begin with the diagnosis of a malignant disease and initial treatment and continue with the aggressive use of high doses of radiation and chemotherapy employed in BMT. Long-term sequelae following BMT include pulmonary damage, cataracts, oral complications, neurological difficulties relapse, second malignancies, and chronic GVHD. Sequelae in children include growth retardation and endocrine dysfunction and in females, sterility and early menopause.

Long-term effects of BMT on the pulmonary system include both restrictive and obstructive disease. Clark and colleagues found that less than 20% of survivors of BMT developed restrictive lung disease as evidenced by a decrease in total lung capacity at one year post-transplant (Clark et al., 1987). Less than 10% of BMT survivors without chronic GVHD develop obstructive pulmonary disease 6 to 12 months following transplant (Clark et al., 1987). The cause of obstructive lung disease is unknown. Individuals may respond to treatment with immunosuppressants. Cataract development is seen following BMT and is caused by both the conditioning regimen and the use of steroids. The incidence of cataract formation following single-dose total-body irradiation (TBI) approached 80% and has been reduced to approximately 20% with the use of fractionated TBI (Deeg, 1990). Increases in dental caries are seen following BMT as a result of radiation-induced xerostomia. Children are at risk for developing enamel hypoplasia, arrested root development, premature apical closure, and microdontia (Dahllof, Heimdahl, Bolme, Lonnqvist, & Ringden, 1988) following TBI. These effects are more pronounced in children treated under the age of 6 (Dahllof et al., 1988). Education regarding the nature of these problems is essential, and more frequent visits to the dentist are required. Sugar-free chewing gum may stimulate salivary flow and alleviate the dry mouth associated with xerostomia.

Leukoencephalopathy infrequently occurs following marrow transplantation. Neuropsychological function in children given TBI was studied by McGuire and others using the Wechsler Intelligence Test for Children-Revised and the Wide Range Achievement Test-Revised. Testing was done before transplant and during follow-up visits 1 through 12 years post-transplant. Learning difficulties in reading, spelling, and arithmetic were more likely to occur in younger children and with higher doses of TBI (McGuire, Sanders, Hill, Buckner, & Sullivan, 1991). In a study of 30 adult BMT recipients, cognitive dysfunction in the form of slowed reaction time, reduced attention span and concentration, and reasoning and problem-solving difficulties were reported (Andrykowski et al., 1990). Identifying children at high risk for compromised intellectual development allows the opportunity to develop educational strategies to maximize the child's potential. Developing strategies for dealing with decreased ability to concentrate and a short attention span will empower the patient to regain a sense of control.

Relapse of the underlying malignancy and occurrence of second malignancies related to the conditioning regimen and immunosuppressive therapy represent other difficult problems. Presently there are no known curative therapies available for recipients who relapse following transplant. The disease can be controlled for a period of time with therapy, but quality-of-life issues surrounding any additional treatment must be thoroughly addressed. In the future, as more knowledge and experience are gained, perhaps there will be ways to decrease relapse rates by capitalizing on the GVL effect mentioned earlier or employing other immunomodulatory therapies. The Seattle Transplant Group recently analyzed the incidence of second malignancies in 1,926 patients treated with radiation and chemotherapy and in 320 patients treated with chemotherapy only. Thirty-five of these individuals developed a second cancer occurring from 1½ months to 14 years following transplant. Non-Hodgkin's lymphoma, leukemia, and solid tumors were observed. The incidence of second cancers in this group is 6.69 times higher than that in age-adjusted controls (Witherspoon et al., 1989).

Growth and development, puberty, and endocrine function may be altered as a result of the conditioning regimen. Thyroid function is rarely affected in those children transplanted following a conditioning regimen containing chemotherapy only. For those children transplanted following TBI, the incidence of compensated hypothyroidism ranges from 12 to 56%, and the incidence of overt hypothyroidism ranges from 3 to 13% (Sanders et al., 1989). The wide range in incidence is accounted for by the difference in the delivery of the TBI, with those receiving single-dose TBI at higher risk for thyroid dysfunction than those receiving fractionated doses. Current recommendations are for those individuals with both clinical and subclinical hypothyroidism to receive supplemental hormone therapy (Sanders et al., 1989). TBI, especially when administered as a single dose, is implicated in deficient growth-hormone production, occurring in 40 to 55% of children (Deeg, 1992). Growth velocity in children is affected not only by the decreased levels of growth hormone, but also by the direct effects of TBI on the bones. Borgstrom and Bolme (1988) reported that, 3 years following transplant, 67% of children were one standard deviation or more below their predicted growth curves. Deficiencies of growth hormone have not been observed in children conditioned for transplant with chemotherapy alone (Deeg, 1990). Administration of growth hormone maximizes the child's potential growth following BMT. Following preparation for BMT with single-agent chemotherapy, most boys and girls will experience normal pubertal development. Leydig-cell dysfunction and ovarian failure secondary to TBI causes the onset of puberty to be delayed or not occur at all in both male and female children (Borgstrom & Bolme, 1988). Development of secondary sex characteristics is compromised in 43% of children following TBI, and hormonal therapy is therefore indicated (Sanders et al., 1989).

Sterility is a devastating consequence of BMT. If chemotherapy only is used in preparation for transplant, the age of the female becomes an important determinant in preserving ovarian function. Women under the age of 26 years, treated with single-agent chemotherapy, may recover only ovarian function. In men receiving single-agent chemotherapy, 65% had a return of sperm production and normal hormone levels (Sanders et al., 1989). For both men and women receiving TBI, infertility is almost 100% certain. Leydig-cell function and the production of luteinizing hormone and testosterone are usually normal in men following TBI. However, recovery of spermatogenesis is extremely rare. The majority of women receiving TBI will have permanent ovarian failure and the onset of premature menopause (Sanders et al., 1989). Counseling individuals pretransplant regarding the options for sperm banking or the storage of fertilized eggs will allow some the opportunity to overcome the devastating effect of sterility following BMT.

TBI causes premature menopause. Symptoms of menopause include vaginitis, insomnia, irritability, vaginal atrophy, osteoporosis, hot flashes, and decreased libido, all of which can interfere with sexual satisfaction post-BMT. Hormone replacement therapy is recommended. Menopause, chemotherapy, and total body irradiation all may cause vaginal dryness. Nurses need to advise women on the nature of this treatment side effect and offer alternatives for vaginal lubrication.

DELAYED EFFECTS OF SOLID ORGAN TRANSPLANTATION

Cardiovascular Problems

Coronary artery disease is a leading cause of death in renal transplant recipients. Risk factors include hypertension, diabetes, smoking, peripheral vascular disease, and hyperlipidemia. The cause of hypertension, which affects 50% of kidney transplant patients (Fabrega, Lopez-Boado, & Gonzalez, 1990), is multifactorial and includes the native kidneys, use of CsA and corticosteroids, graft rejection, poor graft function, and renal artery stenosis (RAS) (Harasyko, 1989). Renin secretion by the native kidneys is a significant contributor to the hypertension observed in renal transplant recipients. Treatment of hypertension may consist of some combination of lowered dosages or withdrawal of corticosteroids, substituting azathioprine, sodium restrictions, antihypertensives, and surgical removal of the native kidneys. The clinician must exercise caution in treating the multifactorial hypertension because correction of one cause may create deleterious effects in graft function or risk an episode of rejection. RAS is a narrowing of the renal artery leading to decreased blood flow to the kidney. The incidence approaches 10% within the first year post-transplant (Fabrega et al., 1990). Ischemic changes occur, leading to hypertension and decreased kidney function. In one series, 20% of diabetic kidney transplant patients and 4% of nondiabetic kidney transplant patients experienced thromboembolic complications during the first year post-transplant (Arnadottir et al., 1983). Diabetes, CsA, and post-transplant erythrocytosis (PTE) may contribute to thromboembolitic complications. PTE is an abnormal rise in hemoglobin of unclear etiology that most frequently develops within the first year following transplant (Fabrega et al., 1990). Anticoagulation therapy is necessary once a diagnosis is established.

Hyperlipidemia is a multifactorial problem that significantly contributes to the incidence of cardiovascular disease in kidney transplant recipients. Risk factors for hyperlipidemia include diabetes, male gender, age, steroid use, obesity, and antihypertensive medications (Pirsch et al., 1992). Increased triglycerides and cholesterol are characteristic of the hyperlipidemia seen in renal graft recipients. Treatment of hyperlipidemia may improve long-term survival of kidney transplant patients by decreasing the mortality associated with cardiovascular disease. Treatment options include withdrawal of corticosteroids as an immunosuppressive agent, use of cholesterol-lowering medications, diet modifications, and weight control (Pirsch et al., 1992). During recovery following kidney transplant, nurses are in a position to help patients minimize the risks associated with the development of coronary artery disease. Diet modifications, exercise programs, and smoking-cessation programs may be useful in decreasing the risks.

Gastrointestinal Problems

Problems of the colon, peptic ulcer disease (PUD), and pancreatitis are all observed following kidney transplant. The incidence of PUD within the first year post-transplant in one series of 1,734 renal transplant patients was 7%, of which 5% developed hemorrhage (Feduska et al., 1984). Factors contributing to PUD include the use of corticosteroids, sepsis, and hepatitis. Aggressive prophylactic use of antacids is recommended. During the first 3 months following transplant, when the doses of immunosuppressive therapy are highest, is the time of greatest risk for perforation and bleeding of the colon. Although the incidence is only 1 to 2%, this complication carries a high mortality. Treatment strategies include early diagnosis and reduction or discontinuation of immunosuppressant agents, antibiotic therapy, and surgical intervention (Fabrega et al., 1990). Viral infections in this population may also contribute to GI problems, particularly CMV infection, which was noted earlier. Hypercalcemia, lipid abnormalities, and viruses play a role in the development of pancreatitis, which occurs in less than 5% of patients and is associated with a high mortality (Fabrega et al., 1990).

Hepatic Disease

Chronic hepatitis, infections, medications, and alcohol use all contribute to liver dysfunction following kidney transplant. Six percent of kidney transplant patients died as a result of liver failure secondary to the hepatitis B virus in one series (LeFrancois et al., 1987). Monitoring for hepatitis antigens, immunization with the hepatitis B vaccine, using the lowest dose possible of immunosuppressive medications, and prescreening transplant candidates for active alcoholism are strategies for decreasing the incidence of liver dysfunction.

Bone Disease

Bone disease in the form of osteonecrosis is a disabling problem faced by 10% of renal transplant recipients (Warner, Karas, & Thornhill, 1988). Osteonecrosis is the death of cellular elements of the bone, which eventually causes bony collapse and primarily affects the femoral head (Fabrega et al., 1990). Use of corticosteroids is a significant risk factor, although the cause is multifactorial. Younger patients are often affected, and bilateral involvement is common. Pain in the involved joint or joints is usually the first warning and often precedes radiographic changes. Prevention includes efforts during the pretransplant dialysis period to protect the bones, early transplantation, and employing low-maintenance doses of corticosteroids.

Long-term sequelae in the cardiac transplant population are primarily due to the effects of life-long immunosuppression and include osteoporosis, diabetes, visual disorders, musculoskeletal disorders, and malignancies (Rosenblum, Rosen, Pine, Rosen, & Borg-Sarin, 1993). Problems faced by other organ recipients are also primarily due to chronic immunosuppressive therapy.

MALIGNANCIES

The incidence of malignancy in organ recipients is approximately 5% (Sheil, Disney, Mathew, Amiss, & Excell, 1991). Compared to age-matched controls, a threefold higher incidence of cancer is reported in transplant recipients (Kinlen, 1985). The most common malignancies that occur are squamous cell carcinomas, non-Hodgkin's lymphoma (NHL) or lymphoproliferative disorders, Kaposi's sarcoma (KS), uterine cancer, and carcinomas of the vulva and perineum. This is in contrast to the most commonly occurring cancers in the United States, which are lung, breast, colorectal, and prostate. Malignancies occurring in immunosuppressed individuals demonstrate a variety of features that are distinctly different from the same malignancy arising in age-matched controls. The development of malignancies associated with immunosuppressive therapy is key information the transplant recipient must receive pretransplant during the informed consent process. Nurses must take an active role in developing screening programs for the early detection of malignancies as part of ongoing follow-up in the post-transplant phase.

Cancers of the skin and lip are most common. The most frequent histology is squamous cell carcinoma, in contrast to the nonimmunosuppressed individual, in whom the most common histology is basal cell carcinoma. This skin cancer typically presents with multiple lesions and is more likely to metastasize compared to the same malignancy in nonimmunosuppressed individuals (Penn, 1988b). In a series of long-term survivors of kidney transplant, Lee and others report that 17 of 20 patients experienced skin lesions. Half of these were malignant squamous cell carcinoma that responded to local therapy (Lee, Posner, King, Brown, & Reams, 1993). In one multicenter study, 42 cases of NHL were observed in renal transplant recipients compared to an expected occurrence rate of 0.85 in the general population (Kinlen, 1985).

Characteristics that differ from NHL in the general population include a predilection for extranodal disease (73%), particularly the central nervous system (33%) (Penn, 1988a). The Epstein-Barr virus genome is almost always found in the involved tissue and considered to be an important factor in the development of post-transplant lymphomas (Nalesnik, Demetris, Fung, & Starzl, 1991). Withdrawal of immunosuppressive therapy often causes spontaneous regression of the lymphoma, and many times the graft will not be lost to rejection (Starzl et al., 1984). Other forms of treatment include the use of acyclovir, cytotoxic chemotherapy, and surgical resection (Nalesnik et al., 1988; Starzl et al., 1984). KS is frequently recognized as a tumor associated with immunosuppression or in those infected with the human immunodeficiency virus (HIV). In renal transplant patients, the incidence of KS is 400- to-500-fold higher than in age-matched controls (Kinlen, 1985). In patients with localized disease, 50% achieved a remission; and in almost half of those achieving remission, the only therapy was a reduction in immunosuppressive therapy (Penn, 1986). Carcinomas of the uterine cervix, vulva, and perineum also occurred much more frequently in transplant recipients than in age-matched controls. Many of these are discovered as carcinoma in situ, which respond to surgical excision (Penn, 1988b). Penn proposed the following as explanations for the development of malignancies secondary to immunosuppression (Penn, 1986, pp. 603–610):

1. Immunosuppressive therapy weakens the immune system's ability to identify, destroy, and remove carcinogens.
2. Antigenic stimulation and activation of oncogenic viruses may play a role.

3. Immunosuppressive treatment may potentiate the effects of carcinogens.

The following is a review of several studies that evaluate the incidence of malignancy post-transplant in relationship to the immunosuppressive therapy utilized. This evaluation must continue as new immunosuppressive therapies emerge. Frei and colleagues looked at the incidence of malignancies in 1,620 kidney transplant patients performed between 1981 and 1991. The maintenance immunosuppressive protocol included CsA and prednisone at a dosage of 7.5mg/day. Episodes of rejection were treated with higher dosages of steroids or in 7% of patients with antilymphocytic sera. Sixty-six malignancies were detected, the most frequent being skin cancer. The risk in this group of developing a malignancy within 10 years is 13.5% (Frei et al., 1993).

In an effort to determine if the pattern of malignancies in kidney transplant patients was shifting with the use of CsA, Gruber and colleagues studied 2,030 kidney recipients who did not receive CsA immunosuppression and 1,317 kidney recipients who did receive CsA. They found no statistically significant differences in cancer incidence between the two groups (Gruber et al., 1991). Efforts are being made to identify subsets of renal graft recipients at highest risk for the development of lymphoproliferative disease following transplant. Three Canadian transplant centers completed a retrospective analysis of seven patients who developed NHL shortly after transplant. They identified the following risk factors: primary EBV infection, induction and anti-rejection therapy with both antilymphocyte globulin (ALG) and OKT3 sequentially, and mismatched EBV grafts (Cockfield et al., 1991). Swinnen and colleagues did a retrospective analysis of 154 heart transplants performed at Loyola University between 1984 and 1990. They found the incidence of lymphoproliferative disorders to be ninefold higher in the group that received OKT3. A statistically significant ($P < 0.001$) higher incidence of lymphoproliferative malignancy was noted in recipients who received a cumulative dose of OKT3 of greater than 75 mg (Swinnen et al., 1990). Other striking features of this analysis were the rapid onset, occurring 1 to 2 months post-transplant, and the aggressive nature of these malignancies.

It is known that cancer may be transmitted from the donor organ to the recipient. Penn reviewed 113 cases reported to the Cincinnati Transplant Tumor Registry up to the end of 1987 (Penn, 1988b). Careful screening and selection of donors is the key to preventing this transmission, which is indeed a rare event in light of the number of organ transplants currently being performed.

LIFE FOLLOWING TRANSPLANT

Despite what appears to be a long and overwhelming list of complications following transplantation, most recipients report an improved quality of life (QOL). This area of study is relatively new and is an area rich in opportunities for nursing. What outcomes need to be addressed and studied to determine the factors that influence the recovery and rehabilitation of the transplant recipients is an area desperately needing clarification and consensus. Nurses involved in transplant care are in a key position to initiate and coordinate long-term follow-up to identify, quantify, describe, and develop interventions to minimize the long-term sequelae associated with transplantation.

Employment

Kinnaert and colleagues report that 55% of patients on hemodialysis work full-time and 53% of kidney transplant recipients work full-time (Kinnaert, Vereerstraeten, & Toussaint, 1985). This has been disappointing to many in the field, who assumed that individuals freed from the daily ritual of dialysis would return to full-time employment. Even more noteworthy in this study was that 83% of those not working following kidney transplant were judged by the medical group as capable of returning to work (Kinnaert et al., 1985). In a series of 24 patients surviving over 20 years following kidney transplantation, 16 are employed and 7 are retired (Fehrman-Ekholm, Gabel, Persson, & Backman, 1993). In one series, 44% of cardiac recipients were unemployed, but only 8% considered themselves unable to find employment (Rosenblum, Rosen, Pine, Rosen, & Borg-Sarin, 1993). The QOL scores as measured by the Sickness Impact Scale in this group were significantly higher in those who returned to work (Rosenblum et al., 1993). Similarly, in a series of 250 cardiac transplant patients reported by Paris and others, 45% were employed, 36% were unemployed, 13% were medically disabled, and 6% retired (Paris et al., 1993). This study looked at variables that might predict who returned to work and under what circumstances. They report the following factors influencing who returned to work following cardiac transplant: the patient's perception of being able to work, no loss of health insurance or disability income, an education level of greater than 12 years, a longer period of time between transplant and the return to work, and a shorter period of disability pretransplant.

Like the series reported by Kinnaert and others in kidney transplant recipients, there was a substantial number of cardiac transplant patients who were not working posttransplant who were judged capable of working by the transplant team. Craven and others reported on the functional outcome and satisfaction of lung transplant recipients (Craven, Bright, & Dear, 1990). Fifty-five percent returned to work with 32% returning full time. However, 64% reported that their physical health limited their ability to work to some extent (Craven et al., 1990). Approximately 35-40% of liver transplant patients returned to full- or part-time employment, with approximately 40% on disability (Knechtle et al., 1993). Schmidt and others reported that, in a study of 212 BMT recipients, 74% returned to full- or part-time work or school and 26% did not return to work or school. They also reported that 90% of pediatric BMT recipients attending school pretransplant returned to school or work (Schmidt et al., 1993).

There are several directions for transplant teams to take to improve the rate of return to gainful employment. One is a more integrated rehabilitation program following transplant to include vocational retraining and education. This is especially true in individuals with less than 12 years' education, blue-collar jobs, and long periods of pretransplant disability. Another is to work to ensure legislation that does not penalize those who wish to return to work by creating financial loss through a reduction or loss in health insurance or disability income. Certainly systems can be devised that can complement gainful employment rather than discourage it. Psychological counseling may be helpful for patients who perceive they are unable to work by helping them discover a more positive image of themselves. Transplant team members need to approach the issues surrounding employment early in the pretransplant phase as a realistic and expected goal following recovery. It is not surprising that a return to work is associated with improved reports of life satisfaction in most transplant recipients.

Individuals who have received organ transplants are disabled according to the definitions contained in the 1990 Americans with Disabilities Act (ADA). These laws were put into place to provide protection against discrimination to those with disabilities. Issues for employers who hire the immunocompromised are only now being addressed (Behling & Guy, 1993). Transplant recipients need regular medical follow-up and need to take time off work for visits to the transplant center. It is important to keep in mind that for many patients this will require traveling to a center that may be a distance from their home. The ADA states that employers need to make allowances for time away from work. For smaller companies, this can create a negative impact on other employees' work schedules, productivity, and deadlines. Issues related to confidentiality in the work place will arise. Businesses are also faced with rising insurance costs for their employees, and transplant recipients require life-long medical care that includes at the very least expensive immunosuppressive medications. Issues surrounding liability if an immunocompromised patient contacts an illness or infection at work have not been sorted out (Behling & Guy, 1993). The ADA states that employers need to make reasonable modifications to the work place to accommodate those with disabilities. What accommodations may be done to decrease the risks of infection posed to the immunosuppressed employee is unclear. There are currently many issues regarding the employment of the transplant recipient that will need to be addressed in the very near future. As patient advocates, nurses can take an active role in helping educate legislative representatives on these complex issues.

Sexual Satisfaction

In a study by Kinnaert, 34% of patients following kidney transplant reported a decrease or absence of sexual activity, compared to 66% of patients on hemodialysis. Patients less than 30 years of age reported the most improvement (Kinnaert et al., 1985). Sixty-five percent of 157 adult BMT survivors reported sexual satisfaction following transplant (Wingard, Curbow, Baker, Zabora, & Piantadosi, 1992). Twenty-two percent of patients in this study reported sexual dissatisfaction. Men in this survey reported difficulties with erection (24%) and ejaculation (13%) as factors associated with sexual dissatisfaction. No physiologic reason for these difficulties was determined. All of the 43 men tested had normal serum testosterone levels. For the women in this study, the loss of menses was reported to be associated with sexual dissatisfaction. Fifty percent of women who did not have a monthly menstrual cycle reported sexual satisfaction, compared to 80% with a monthly menstrual cycle. Further analysis revealed that the following factors were associated with positive sexual satisfaction: younger age, a diagnosis of aplastic anemia, positive feelings regarding their appearance, overall satisfaction with life, and a satisfying relationship with their significant other. An interesting finding of this analysis was that no correlation between sexual satisfaction pre-transplant and post-transplant was found (Wingard et al., 1992). In a study of 212 BMT recipients, 69% reported their sexual activity to be similar to prediagnosis, and 15% reported that their sexual activity was less than prediagnosis levels (Schmidt et al., 1993).

As mentioned earlier, menopause can also contribute to sexual dissatisfaction in women post-BMT. These studies illustrate the need for nurses to assess transplant recipients actively during recovery to identify those individuals with decreased sexual satisfaction. Providing an opportunity for the patient and partner to discuss these issues is an important role for nurses to play in the recovery of transplant recipients. Open and honest discussions with the patient and partner can help bridge communication and alleviate fears and anxiety. Due to the sensitive nature of these problems, patients are often reluctant to initiate this discussion with members of the health care team. Nurses who have established a trusting relationship are in a unique position to address these sensitive and important concerns.

Quality of Life

Quality of life (QOL) is emerging as an important component for evaluating successful outcome of therapy. It has become important in all areas of medicine to move beyond survival data and incorporate parameters of success as defined by the survivor. QOL is a multidimensional concept, and determining what domains to investigate to answer the question "What is the transplant recipient's QOL?" is a difficult task. QOL studies are complicated by a number of problems, including the lack of a standardized definition of QOL, lack of validated tools, the subjective nature of the question, absence of culturally diverse tools, and agreement as to what variables are important. Despite these problems, many attempts have been made to evaluate QOL in transplant recipients. Most studies look at some combination of physical, emotional, psychosocial, and global components. Recovery challenges for transplant recipients are numerous and include returning to work. For some, this may be following an extensive period of disability pretransplant. Other challenges are posed by the resumption of prior roles and responsibilities; coping with changes in body image; dealing with the side effects of the immunosuppressive therapy; and coping with the ongoing threat of rejection, chronic GVHD, and in some cases relapse of the underlying condition. Emotional difficulties post-transplant include anxiety, depression, body-image disturbances, mood alterations, family stress, and sleep disturbances. Long-term studies of the coping and adaptation of transplant survivors and their families are needed in order to develop strategies to facilitate a healthy adaptation posttransplant.

In general, it is reported that most patients report improved quality of life following transplant. Evans and colleagues compared QOL in cardiac and kidney transplant patients to those patients receiving dialysis and the general population (Evans, Manninen, Maier, Garrison, & Hart, 1985). On measures of well-being, kidney transplant patients scored highest at 11.83 (range of 2.1 to 14.7), followed by the general population and cardiac transplant patients. The lowest scores were reported for dialysis patients.

The Index of Well-Being is a combined score using the Overall Life Satisfaction and the Index of Psychological Affect. Life satisfaction scores were also highest in kidney transplant patients followed by the general population and dialysis patients, and the lowest scores were found in cardiac transplant recipients. This study by Evans and colleagues was a descriptive study only, and no statistical analysis was done (Evans et al., 1985). In lung transplant recipients, 72% reported their physical health to be good to excellent, 86% reported their emotional health to be good to excellent, and 73% reported life satisfaction be good to excellent (Craven et al., 1990). In cardiac recipients, QOL scores obtained using the Sickness Impact Scale were lower than in the general population, similar to cardiac arrest patients and better than individuals with low back pain (Rosenblum et al., 1993). In a large QOL study by Schmidt and others, BMT recipients were asked to rate their QOL on a linear analog scale of 1 to 10, with 1 being the lowest QOL and 10 being the highest. Seventy-eight percent of adults rated their QOL greater than or equal to 8. The vast majority of patients in this study reported positive feelings regarding their appearance and a normal-to- excellent appetite. Twenty-three percent of adults and 14% of children rated their sleeping patterns as variable to poor. Factors that impacted negatively on QOL scores included sexual dissatisfaction and the need for regular medication. Eighty-seven percent of subjects in this study remained married following transplant (Schmidt et al., 1993).

As the number of survivors of all forms of transplantation increase, the issues surrounding recovery, immunosuppressive therapy, adaptation, family stress, financial security, rehabilitation and other QOL issues become more important than ever. Nurses can take a lead in designing studies to identify and develop strategies to overcome the long-term health consequences, both physical and emotional, of transplant recipients. Further nursing research is needed in many areas addressed in this chapter (see Table 4.4).

TABLE 4.4 Ideas for Future Nursing Research

- Facilitating compliance with immunosuppressive therapies
- Decreasing the side effects of immunosuppressive therapies
- Measuring understanding of treatment risks and benefits
- Defining QOL and the domains to be studied
- Developing validated, reliable, and culturally sensitive QOL tools
- Designing studies of adaptation and coping for patients and families
- Validating strategies to facilitate understanding and coping

CONCLUSION

It is imperative that each nurse working within the challenging and exciting field of transplantation understand fully the effects that such aggressive therapies have on the long-term health and well-being of the patients they serve. As technology allows us to save and restore the health of many more individuals, we need to ask ourselves constantly, "What is the quality of the life they lead following these treatments?" A small decrease in chronic graft rejection at the cost of severe impact on the patient's functional status or increased risk of malignancy may not be advantageous in the long run. Curing patients and not enabling them to return to their employment and other social roles is inadequate. Counseling and rehabilitation begin with the initial consult for treatment and continue throughout the long trajectory of recovery.

Addressing not only the physical issues, but also the psychological issues, faced by transplant recipients requires a comprehensive transplant program that can address the challenges faced by transplant recipients and their families throughout the transplant experience. Many questions remain regarding the long-term impact of transplantation, and the field is rich with opportunities for nursing research. If it is imperative to begin counseling and rehabilitation during the initial consult with the transplant team, how can we provide the information in a way that is heard and understood? Much needs to be examined and understood before the interventions we undertake will impact positively on the recovery transplant recipients. Much of this work has begun, and we must continue the momentum. Transplantation is a field that is sure to grow with the coming decades.

REFERENCES

Adams, D. H., & Tilney, N. L. (1989). The pathobiology of chronic rejection. *Transplant Review, 3,* 131–152.

Anderson, B. A., Young, P. V., Kean, W. F., Ludwin, S. K., Galbraith, P. R., & Anastassiades, T. P. (1982). Polymyositis in chronic graft vs host disease: A case report. *Archives of Neurology, 39,* 188–190.

Andrykowski, M. A., Altmaier, E. M., Barnett, R. L., Burish, T. G., Gingrich, R., & Henslee-Downey, P. J. (1990). Cognitive dysfunction in adult survivors of allogeneic marrow transplantation: Relationship to dose of total body irradiation. *Bone Marrow Transplantation, 6,* 269–276.

Arnadottir, M., Bergentz, S. E., Bergqvist, D., Husberg, B., Konrad, P., & Lindholm, T. (1983). Thromboembolic complications after renal transplantation: A retrospective analysis. *World Journal of Surgery, 7,* 757–761.

Arvin, A. M. (1993). Herpes virus infection after marrow transplantation. *Marrow Transplantation Reviews, 3,* 29–31.

Atkinson, K. (1990). Chronic graft-versus-host disease. *Bone Marrow Transplantation, 5,* 69–82.

Atkinson, K. (1992). Chronic graft-versus-host disease following marrow transplantation. *Marrow Transplantation Reviews, 2,* 1–7.

Atkinson, K., Horowitz, M. M., Gale, R. P., van Bekkum, D. W., Gluckman, E., Good, R. A., Jacobsen, N., Kolb, H. J., Rimm, A. A., Ringden, O., Rozman, C., Sobocinski, K. A., Zwaan, F. E., & Bortin, M. M. (1990). Risk factors for chronic graft-versus-host disease after HLA-identical sibling bone marrow transplantation. *Blood, 75,* 2459–2464.

Atkinson, K., Storb, R., Prentice, R. L., Weiden, P. L., Witherspoon, R. P., Sullivan, K., Noel, D., & Thomas, E. D. (1979). Analysis of late infections in 89 long-term survivors of bone marrow transplantation. *Blood, 53,* 720–731.

Atkinson, K., Weller, P., Ryman, W., & Biggs, J. (1986). PUVA therapy for drug-resistant graft-versus-host disease. *Bone Marrow Transplantation, 1,* 227–236.

Behling, D., & Guy, J. (1993). Who's protected? Legal, ethical issues in employing the immunosuppressed. *Occupational Health & Safety, 62,* 76–79.

Blume, K. G., & Chao, N. J. (1992). Surviving the cure. *Marrow Transplantation Reviews, 2,* 14–15.

Bolger, G. B., Sullivan, K. M., Spence, A. M., Appelbaum, F. R., Johnston, R., Sanders, J. E., Deeg, H. J., Witherspoon, R. P., Doney, K. C., Nims, J., Thomas, E. D., & Storb, R. (1986). Myasthenia gravis after allogeneic bone marrow transplantation: Relationship to chronic graft-versus-host disease. *Neurology, 36,* 1087–1091.

Borgstrom, B., & Bolme, P. (1988). Studies of the endocrine system in children after allogeneic bone marrow transplantation. *Bone Marrow Transplantation, 3*(Suppl. 1), 261–262.

Bortin, M. M., Horowitz, M. M., & Rimm, A. A. (1992). Progress report from the International Bone Marrow Transplant Registry. *Bone Marrow Transplantation, 10,* 113–122.

Chao, N. J. (1992). Graft versus host disease following allogeneic bone marrow transplantation. *Current Opinion in Immunology, 4,* 571–576.

Chao, N. J. (1994). *Graft-versus-host disease.* Austin: R. G. Landes Company.

Clark, J. G., Schwartz, D. A., Flournoy, N., Sullivan, K. M., Crawford, S. W., & Thomas, E. D. (1987). Risk factors for airflow obstruction in recipients of bone marrow transplants. *Annals of Internal Medicine, 107,* 648–656.

Cockfield, S. M., Preiksaitis, J., Harvey, E., Jones, C., Hebert, D., Keown, P., & Halloran, P. F. (1991). Is sequential use of ALG and OKT3 in renal transplants associated with an increased incidence of fulminant posttransplant lymphoproliferative disorder? *Transplantation Proceedings, 23,* 1106–1107.

Craven, J. L., Bright, J., & Dear, C. L. (1990). Psychiatric, psychosocial, and rehabilitative aspects of lung transplantation. *Clinics in Chest Medicine, 11,* 247–257.

Dahllof, G., Barr, M., Bolme, P., Modeer, T., Lonnqvist, B., Ringden, O., & Heimdahl, A. (1988). Disturbances in dental development after total body irradiation in bone marrow transplant recipients. *Oral Surgery Oral Medicine and Oral Pathology, 65,* 41–44.

Dahllof, G., Heimdahl, A., Bolme, P., Lonnqvist, B., & Ringden, O. (1988). Oral condition in children treated with bone marrow transplantation. *Bone Marrow Transplantation, 3,* 43–51.

Deeg, H. J. (1990). Delayed complications and long-term effects after bone marrow transplantation. *Hematology/Oncology Clinics of North America, 4,* 641–657.

Deeg, H. J. (1992). Delayed complications of marrow transplantation. *Marrow Transplantation Reviews, 2,* 10–13.

Dunn, D. L. (1990). Problems related to immunosuppression. *Critical Care Clinics, 6,* 955–977.

Evans, R. W., Manninen, D. L., Maier, A., Garrison, L. P., & Hart, L. G. (1985). The quality of life of kidney and heart transplant recipients. *Transplantation Proceedings, 17,* 1579–1582.

Fabrega, A. J., Lopez-Boado, M., & Gonzalez, S. (1990). Problems in the long-term renal allograft recipient. *Critical Care Clinics, 6,* 979–1005.

Feduska, N. J., Amend, W. J. C., Vincenti, F., Melzer, J. S., Duca, R., Garovoy, M. R., & Salvatierra, O. (1984). Peptic ulcer disease in kidney transplant recipients. *The American Journal of Surgery, 148,* 51–57.

Fehrman-Ekholm, I., Gabel, H., Persson, N. H., & Backman, U. (1993). Characteristics of long-term survivors (>20 years) after kidney transplantation. *Transplantation Proceedings, 25,* 1334–1335.

Ferrara, J. L. M., & Deeg, H. J. (1991). Graft-versus-host disease. *The New England Journal of Medicine, 324,* 667–674.

Frei, U., Bode, U., Repp, H., Schindler, R., Brunkhorst, R., Vogt, P., Hauss, J., & Pichlmayr, R. (1993). Malignancies under cyclosporine after kidney transplantation: Analysis of a 10-year period. *Transplantation Proceedings, 25,* 1394–1396.

Gao, S. Z., Schroeder, J. S., Alderman, E. L., Hunt, S. A., Valantine, H. A., Wiederhold, V., & Stinson, E. B. (1989). Prevalence of accelerated coronary artery disease in heart transplant survivors. *Circulation, 80*(Suppl. 3), 100–105.

Gao, S. Z., Schroeder, J. S., Hunt, S., & Stinson, E. B. (1988). Retransplantation for severe accelerated coronary artery disease in heart transplant recipients. *The American Journal of Cardiology, 62,* 876–881.

Gomez-Garcia, P., Herrera-Arroyo, C., Torres-Gomez, A., Gomez-Carrasco, J., Aljama-Garcia, P., Lopez-Rubio, F., Martinez-Guibelalde, F., Fornes-Torres, G., & Rojas-Contreras, R. (1988). Renal involvement in chronic graft-versus-host disease: A report of two cases. *Bone Marrow Transplantation, 3,* 357–362.

Grattan, M. T., Moreno-Cabral, C. E., Starnes, V. A., Oyer, P. E., Stinson, E. B., & Shumway, N. E. (1989). Cytomegalovirus infection is associated with cardiac allograft rejection and atherosclerosis. *Journal of the American Medical Association, 261,* 3561–3566.

Greenspan, A., Deeg, H. J., Cottler-Fox, M., Sirdofski, M., Spitzer, T. R., & Kattah,

J. (1990). Incapacitating peripheral neuropathy as a manifestation of chronic graft-versus-host disease. *Bone Marrow Transplantation, 5,* 349–353.

Griffith, B. P., Hardesty, R. L., Armitage, J. M., Hattler, B. G., Pham, S. M., Keenan, R. J., & Paradis, I. (1993). A decade of lung transplantation. *Annals of Surgery, 218,* 310–320.

Grond, J., Gouw, A. S. H., Poppema, S., Slooff, M. J. H., & Gips, C. H. (1986). Chronic rejection in liver transplants: A histopathologic analysis of failed grafts and antecedent serial biopsies. *Transplantation Proceedings, 18*(Suppl. 4), 128–135.

Gruber, S. A., Skjei, K. L., Sothern, R. B., Robison, L., Tzardis, P., Moss, A., Gillingham, K., Canafax, D. M., Matas, A. J., & Dunn, D. L. (1991). Cancer development in renal allograft recipients treated with conventional and cyclosporine immunosuppression. *Transplantation Proceedings, 23,* 1104–1105.

Harasyko, C. (1989). Kidney transplantation. *Nursing Clinics of North America, 24,* 851–863.

Holland, H. K., Wingard, J. R., Beschorner, W. E., Saral, R., & Santos, G. W. (1988). Bronchiolitis obliterans in bone marrow transplantation and its relationship to chronic graft-v-host disease and low serum IgG. *Blood, 72,* 621–627.

Horowitz, M. M., Gale, R. P., Sondel, P. M., Goldman, J. M., Kersey, J., Kolb, H. J., Rimm, A. A., Ringden, O., Rozman, C., Speck, B., Truitt, R. L., Zwaan, F. E., & Bortin, M. M. (1990). Graft-versus-leukemia reactions after bone marrow transplantation. *Blood, 75,* 555–562.

Hruban, R. H., Beschorner, W. E., Baumgartner, W. A., Augustine, S. M., Ren, H., Reitz, B. A., & Hutchins, G. M. (1990). Accelerated arteriosclerosis in heart transplant recipients is associated with a t-lymphocyte-mediated endothelialitis. *American Journal of Pathology, 137,* 871–882.

Kerman, R. H., Kimball, P., Scheinen, S., Radovancevic, B., Van Buren, C. T., Kahan, B. D., & Frazier, O. H. (1994). The relationship among donor-recipient HLA mismatches, rejection and death from coronary artery disease in cardiac transplant recipients. *Transplantation, 57,* 884–888.

Kinlen, L. J. (1985). Incidence of cancer in rheumatoid arthritis and other disorders after immunosuppressive treatment. *American Journal of Medicine, 78,* 44–49.

Kinnaert, P., Vereerstraeten, P., & Toussaint, C. (1985). Vocational rehabilitation and sexual behavior after renal transplantation. *Transplantation Proceedings, 17,* 1583–1584.

Knechtle, S. J., Fleming, M. F., Barry, K. L., Steen, D., Pirsch, J. D., D'Alessandro, A. M., Kalayoglu, M., & Belzer, F. O. (1993). Liver transplantation in alcoholics: Assessment of psychological health and work activity. *Transplantation Proceedings, 25,* 1916–1918.

Knobler, H. Y., Sagher, U., Peled, I. J., Wexler, M. R., Steiner, D., Rubinstein, N., Weshler, Z., Or, R., & Slavin, S. (1985). Tolerance to donor-type skin in the recipient of a bone marrow allograft. *Transplantation, 40,* 223–225.

Krowka, M. J., Rosenow, E. C., & Hoagland, H. C. (1985). Pulmonary complications of bone marrow transplantation. *Chest, 87,* 237–246.

Kurzrock, R., Zander, A., Kanojia, M., Vellekoop, L., Spitzer, G., Jagannath, S.,

Schell, S., Peters, L., & Dicke, K. (1984). Obstructive lung disease after allogeneic bone marrow transplantation. *Transplantation, 37,* 156–160.

Land, W. (1989). Kidney transplantation: State of the art. *Transplantation Proceedings, 21,* 1425–1429.

Lee, H. M., Posner, M. P., King, A. L., Brown, K. B., & Reams, D. R. (1993). Status of long-term (25 years) survival of kidney transplant patients. *Transplantation Proceedings, 25,* 1336–1337.

LeFrancois, N., Elmghabbar, N., Chossegros, P., Betuel, H., Faure, J. L., Revillard, J. P., Traeger, J., Dubernard, J. M., & Touraine, J. L. (1987). Long-term results in kidney transplantation: Patient and graft survival, causes of graft failure and mortality, renal function, and complications after 10 years. *Transplantation Proceedings, 19,* 3767–3768.

Ludwig, J., Wiesner, R. H., Batts, K. P., Perkins, J. D., & Krom, R. A. F. (1987). The acute vanishing bile duct syndrome (acute irreversible rejection) after orthotopic liver transplantation. *Hepatology, 7,* 476–483.

Lum, L. G. (1990). Immune recovery after bone marrow transplantation. *Hematology/Oncology Clinics of North America, 4,* 659–675.

McDonald, G. B., Shulman, H. M., Sullivan, K. M., & Spencer, G. D. (1986). Intestinal and hepatic complications of human bone marrow transplantation: Part II. *Gastroenterology, 90,* 770–784.

McGuire, T., Sanders, J. E., Hill, D., Buckner, C. D., & Sullivan, K. M. (1991). Neuropsychological function in children given total body irradiation for marrow transplantation. *Experimental Hematology, 19* (Abstract 462), 578.

Muirhead, J. (1989). Heart and heart-lung transplantation. *Nursing Clinics of North America, 24,* 865–880.

Nalesnik, M. A., Demetris, A. J., Fung, J. J., & Starzl, T. E. (1991). Lymphoproliferative disorders arising under immunosuppression with FK 506: Initial observations in a large transplant population. *Transplantation Proceedings, 23,* 1108–1110.

Nalesnik, M. A., Jaffe, R., Starzl, T. E., Demetris, A. J., Porter, K., Burnham, J. A., Makowka, L., Ho, M., & Locker, J. (1988). The pathology of posttransplant lymphoproliferative disorders occurring in the setting of cyclosporine A-prednisone immunosuppression. *American Journal of Pathology, 133,* 173–192.

Paris, W., Woodbury, A., Thompson, S., Levick, M., Nothegger, S., Arbuckle, P., Hutkin-Slade, L., & Cooper, D. K. C. (1993). Returning to work after heart transplantation. *Journal of Heart and Lung Transplantation, 12,* 46–54.

Penn, I. (1986). Cancer is a complication of severe immunosuppression. *Surgery, Gynecology & Obstetrics, 162,* 603–610.

Penn, I. (1988a). Transmission of cancer with donor organs. *Transplantation Proceedings, 20,* 739–740.

Penn, I. (1988b). Tumors of the immunocompromised patient. *Annual Review of Medicine, 39,* 63–73.

Pillon, L. R. (1991). Cyclosporine: A nursing focus on immunosuppressive therapy. *Dimensions of Critical Care Nursing, 10,* 68–73.

Pirsch, J. D., D'Alessandro, A. M., Sollinger, H. W., Knechtle, S. J., Reed, A.,

Kalayoglu, M., & Belzer, F. O. (1992). Hyperlipidemia and transplantation: Etiologic factors and therapy. *Journal of the American Society of Nephrology, 2*(Suppl. 3), S238–S242.

Quan, C. M., & Bowden, R. A. (1993). Clinical aspects of cytomegalovirus infection in marrow transplantation. *Marrow Transplantation Reviews, 3,* 17–32.

Rhodes, D. F., Lee, W. M., Wingard, J.R., Pavy, M. D., Santos, G. W., Shaw, B. W., Wood, R. P., Sorrell, M. F., & Markin, R. S. (1990). Orthotopic liver transplantation for graft-versus-host disease following bone marrow transplantation. *Gastroenterology, 99,* 536–538.

Rosenblum, D. S., Rosen, M. L., Pine, Z. M., Rosen, S. H., & Borg-Sarin, J. (1993). Health status and quality of life following cardiac transplantation. *Archives of Physical Medicine and Rehabilitation, 74,* 490–493.

Rubin, R. H. (1993). Fungal and bacterial infections in the immunocompromised host. *European Journal of Clinical Microbiology and Infectious Disease, 12*(Suppl 1), S42–S48.

Ruutu, T., Ruutu, M., Volin, L., & Leskinen, R. (1988). Severe cystitis as a manifestation of chronic graft-versus-host disease after bone marrow transplantation. *British Journal of Urology, 62,* 612–613.

Sanders, J., Sullivan, K., Witherspoon, R., Doney, K., Anasetti, C., Beatty, P., & Petersen, F. B. (1989). Long term effects and quality of life in children and adults after marrow transplantation. *Bone Marrow Transplantation, 4*(Suppl. 4), 27–29.

Schmidt, G. M., Niland, J. C., Forman, S. J., Fonbuena, P. P., Dagis, A. C., Grant, M. M., Ferrell, B. R., Barr, T. A., Stallbaum, B. A., Chao, N. J., & Blume, K. G. (1993). Extended follow-up in 212 long-term allogeneic bone marrow transplant survivors. *Transplantation, 55,* 551–557.

Sheets, L. (1989). Liver transplantation. *Nursing Clinics of North America, 24,* 881–889.

Sheil, A. G. R., Disney, A. P. S., Mathew, T. T., Amiss, N., & Excell, L. (1991). Cancer development in cadaveric donor renal allograft recipients treated with azathioprine (AZA) or cyclosporine (CyA) or AZA/CyA. *Transplantation Proceedings, 23,* 1111–1112.

Snydman, D. R., Werner, B. G., Heinze-Lacey, B., Berardi, V. P., Tilney, N. L., Kirkman, R. L., Milford, E. L., Cho, S. I., Bush, H. L., Levey, A. S., Strom, T. B., Carpenter, G. B., Levey, R. H., Harmon, W. E., Zimmerman, C. E., Shapiro, M. E., Steinman, T., LoGerfo, F., Idelson, B., Schroter, G. P. J., Levin, M. J., McIver, J., Leszczynski, J., & Grady, G. F. (1987). Use of cytomegalovirus immune globulin to prevent cytomegalovirus disease in renal-transplant recipients. *The New England Journal of Medicine, 317,* 1049–1054.

Starzl, T. E., Nalesnik, M. A., Porter, K. A., Ho, M., Iwatsuki, S., Griffith, B. P., Rosenthal, J. T., Hakala, T. R., Shaw, B. W., Hardesty, R. L., Atchison, R. W., Jaffe, R., & Bahnson, H. T. (1984). Reversibility of lymphomas and lymphoproliferative lesions developing under cyclosporine-steroid therapy. *Lancet, 1,* 583–587.

Sullivan, K. M. (1986). Acute and chronic graft-versus-host disease in man. *International Journal of Cell Cloning, 4*(Suppl. 1), 42–93.

Sullivan, K. M., Kopecky, K. J., Jocom, J., Fisher, L., Buckner, C. D., Meyers, J. D., Counts, G. W., Bowden, R. A., Petersen, F. B., Witherspoon, R. P., Budinger, M. D., Schwartz, R. S., Appelbaum, F. R., Clift, R. A., Hansen, J. A., Sanders, J. E., Thomas, E. D., & Storb, R. (1990). Immunomodulatory and antimicrobial efficacy of intravenous immunoglobulin in bone marrow transplantation. *The New England Journal of Medicine, 323,* 705–712.

Swinnen, L. J., Nordin-Costanzo, M. R., Fisher, S. G., O'Sullivan, E. J., Johnson, M. R., Heroux, A. L., Dizikes, G. J., Pifarre, R., & Fisher, R. I. (1990). Increased incidence of lymphoproliferative disorder after immunosuppression with the monoclonal antibody OKT3 in cardiac-transplant recipients. *The New England Journal of Medicine, 323,* 1723–1728.

Tilney, N. L., Whitley, D., Diamond, J. R., Kupiec-Weglinski, J. W., & Adams, D. H. (1991). Chronic rejection: An undefined conundrum. *Transplantation, 52,* 389–398.

Vogelsang, G. B., Farmer, E. R., Hess, A. D., Altamonte, V., Beschorner, W. E., Jabs, D. A., Corio, R. I., Levin, L. S., Colvin, O. M., Wingard, J. R., & Santos, G. W. (1992). Thalidomide for the treatment of chronic graft-versus-host disease. *The New England Journal of Medicine, 326,* 1055–1058.

Vogelsang, G. B., & Wagner, J. E. (1990) Graft-versus-host disease. *Hematology/Oncology Clinics of North America, 4,* 625–639.

Warner, J. J. P., Karas, S., & Thornhill, T. S. (1988). Osteonecrosis after renal transplantation. In P. J. Morris & N. L. Tilney (Eds.), *Transplantation Reviews* (pp. 177–205). Philadelphia: W. B. Saunders.

Williams, T. J., Grossman, R. F., & Maurer, J. R. (1990). Long-term functional follow-up of lung transplant recipients. *Clinics in Chest Medicine, 11,* 347–358.

Wingard, J. R. (1993). Infections in allogeneic bone marrow transplant recipients. *Seminars in Oncology, 20*(Suppl. 6), 80–87.

Wingard, J. R., Curbow, B., Baker, F., Zabora, J., & Piantadosi, S. (1992). Sexual satisfaction in survivors of bone marrow transplantation. *Bone Marrow Transplantation, 9,* 185–190.

Wingard, J. R., Piantadosi, S., Vogelsang, G. B., Farmer, E. R., Jabs, D. A., Levin, S., Beschorner, W. E., Cahill, R. A., Miller, D. F., Harrison, D., Saral, R., & Santos, G. W. (1989). Predictors of death from chronic graft-versus-host disease following bone marrow transplant. *Blood, 74,* 1428–1435.

Winston, D. J., Ho, W.G., Champlin, R. E., & Gale, R. P. (1984). Infectious complications of bone marrow transplantation. *Experimental Hematology, 12,* 205–215.

Witherspoon, R. P., Fisher, L. D., Schoch, G., Martin, P., Sullivan, K. M., Sanders, J., Deeg, H. J., Doney, K., Thomas, D., Storb, R., & Thomas, E. D. (1989). Secondary cancers after bone marrow transplantation for leukemia or aplastic anemia. *The New England Journal of Medicine, 321,* 784–789.

Wujcik, D., Ballard, B., & Camp-Sorrell, D. (1994). Selected complications of allogeneic bone marrow transplantation. *Seminars in Oncology Nursing, 10,* 28–41.

PART II

New Frontiers in Immunosuppression

5

CHIMERISM IN TRANSPLANTATION

Nancy L. Stitt, R.N., B.S.N., C.C.R.N.

Organ transplantation has made remarkable progress in the past three decades. Today, more procedures are being perfected with improved transplant technology and broader indications for transplantation. In spite of these advances, transplant teams are faced with the challenge of dealing with the three major causes of recipient mortality: donor shortage, rejection, and infection. This chapter will discuss one specific solution to the problem of rejection.

Transplant research has always been and still is focused on preventing rejection, as demonstrated by the number of immunosuppressant drugs on the market. Other solutions to the problem of rejection are being investigated. One such concept is to create an environment that is "drugfree," one that does not require immunosuppression and/or antibiotics, and one that accepts the transplanted organ. The answer does not appear to lie in the development of stronger drugs. It lies in the development of tolerance or graft acceptance in transplant recipients. The process by which this occurs is referred to as "chimerism," pronounced "chy-mer-ism."

This area of transplantation is perhaps one of the most fascinating and active areas being explored today. In many ways, it is a "back to the future" phenomenon in that theories and drugs that were available to us in earlier years are resurfacing and being re-examined. This chapter will discuss the meaning of chimerism, the development of tolerance through chimerism, its augmentation, and patient education regarding chimerism.

OVERVIEW OF TRANSPLANT IMMUNOLOGY

To facilitate an understanding of chimerism, it is important to review the history of transplantation theories and transplant immunology. This reexamining of the past will give the reader an appreciation of these theories with the potential for future applications.

Bone Marrow Versus Solid Organ Transplantation

The growth of transplantation was grounded in the works of Medawar. This father of transplant immunology is credited with laying the foundation on which most transplant immunology is based. From the works of Medawar and his two principal associates, Billingham and Brent, in the late 1940s and 1950s, stemmed two separate schools of thought regarding transplantation. The bone marrow group and the solid organ group developed divergent clinical requirements and reactions for successful transplantation (see Table 5.1). Bone marrow graft success is related to several factors, including the following:

- Preconditioning with high-dose chemotherapy to ablate the bone marrow
- Human leukocyte antigen (HLA) matching between donor and recipient

Perfect HLA matching allows engraftment—all done in a drug-free state called tolerance (Starzl, Demetris, Trucco et al., 1993). Graft-versus-host disease (GVHD) is common even with major histocompatibility complex matching. In this model, a one-way mixed leukocyte reaction (MLR) occurs in which leukocytes move in one direction out of the bone marrow. Solid organ transplantation encounters cellular movement as well, but it is considered to be a two-way cellular movement organ, called two-way MLR, in which donor cells leave and recipient cells move into the transplanted organ (Starzl, Demetris, Trucco et al., 1993). Initially, efforts to control and stop this migration of cells were thought to be necessary to

TABLE 5.1 Requirements and Reactions in Transplantation

	Bone Marrow	Solid Organ
Preconditioning	Required	Not required
Tissue Matching	Essential	Not essential
Graft Take	Tolerance	Acceptance
Graft Failure	*GVHD	Rejection
**MLR	One-way	Two-way

*Graft-versus-host disease
**Mixed leukocyte reaction

prevent rejection. This concept is perhaps the most important precursor to the development of tolerance or graft acceptance.

Tolerance and Graft Acceptance

Throughout the years, the terms "classical tolerance," i.e., drugfree, and "graft acceptance" have been interchangeably and ambiguously used. The term "tolerance" routinely has been used among bone marrow transplant physicians to define transplant recipients who are drugfree and tolerating their transplanted bone marrow. The term "graft acceptance," most often used by solid organ transplant surgeons, describes transplant recipients who are not rejecting, with or without immunosuppression. It is now thought that all variants or stages of rejection are part of this cell migration process (Starzl, Demetris, Murase et al., 1992). As transplant immunology is further advanced, more precise terminology such as "donor-specific unresponsiveness," in which there is no response, or attack, to the donor organ or tissue, will replace terms such as tolerance and graft acceptance.

THE FOUR STEPS IN UNDERSTANDING CHIMERISM

To understand this dynamic concept of chimerism, four steps need to be addressed: definition, recognition, enhancement, and education.

Step One: Definition of Chimerism

The classical chimera is the mythical creature that is a combination of animal and human, most often represented as the lion-bodied, human-headed sphinx. In architecture, chimeric figures can be found throughout the world, such as the Tower of Chimeras at the Cathedral of Notre Dame. The scientific chimera is any biological system made up of at least two different genetic components, either of the same or different species, thus creating a genetic composite. In transplantation, chimerism occurs when evidence shows that donor cells have left the donor organ and can be found elsewhere in the recipient and that recipient cells can be found in the donor organ.

One of the most important discoveries in chimerism transplant theory was that of defining exactly what type of cells constituted these migrating cells and where they migrated to. Donor cells leaving the solid organ graft and recipient cells entering the donor organ include cells known as passenger leukocytes (Starzl, Demetris, Murase et al., 1992) and are from a distinct family of bone-marrow-derived, antigen-presenting dendritic leukocytes (Steinman, 1991). These dendritic cells are normally distributed throughout the body, including areas such as the interstitia of the kidney, heart, and other organs once thought not to contain immunologically active cells (Steinman, 1991). After transplantation, the movement of these cells is referred to as "cell traffic" or cell migration. In the past, the presence of recipient lymphocytes in donor grafts was thought to equate with rejection. This cellular movement of antigen-presenting cells was thought to be the mechanism of rejection and something to be prevented. This exchange of migratory leukocytes between the transplant and the recipient with the resultant cellular chimerism in both is now thought to be the secret to graft acceptance for all solid organ allografts and has laid the groundwork for reexamination of xenograft acceptance. These recent observations have enlightened transplant immunologists and have ushered in the era of developing alternative therapeutic strategies surrounding rejection and its prevention (Starzl, Demetris, Trucco et al., 1993).

Step Two: Recognition of Chimerism

Chimerism in Kidney Transplantation. Indirect evidence of chimerism was demonstrated as early as 1963, but at that time, the explanation of cellular migration was not obvious. Thirty years ago, the kidney was thought to be a leukocyte-poor organ; therefore, cells from the donor kidney could not possibly migrate into the recipient tissues. Immunological changes, however, did occur in the recipients as demonstrated through exhaustive skin testing using tuberculin, histoplasmin, blastomycin, coccidioidin, mumps, *Candida* and *Trichophyton.* The Colorado kidney transplant team led by Dr. Thomas Starzl found that when skin reactions were positive preoperatively in the donor and negative in the recipients, after transplant, 77% of the recipients demonstrated a positive skin reaction when tested. When this did not occur in the remaining 23%, the kidney transplant failed as a result of rejection (Starzl, Murase, Demetris et al., 1993).

Direct evidence of chimerism appeared in these same patients more than 28 years later. Immunocytochemical testing, also called cytostaining, and polymerase chain reaction (PCR) are two techniques used to detect chimerism. Cytostaining with HLA monoclonal antibodies allows for the location and morphological characterization of phenotypically distinct donor and recipient cells. PCR distinguishes donor DNA from recipient DNA (using the Y chromosome for male donor-female recipient transplants and/or chromosome 6). Skin, lymph nodes, kidney allograft biopsies, and blood were tested for chimerism. Five kidney transplant recipients from the 1963 Colorado era were selected to be tested for chimerism in 1992. These recipients were selected because four of the living-related donors were still alive, thus allowing for donor HLA retyping and use of their leukocytes for immunocompetence testing of the recipients. The fifth deceased donor was a father-to-daughter donor allowing for sex-typing in the recipient tissue. One of these five recipients had stopped immunosuppression, whereas the remaining four were still taking azathioprine with or without prednisone. Direct evidence of chimerism was shown: donor graft cells were found in the lymph node, skin biopsies and/or blood of the recipients, and the kidney biopsies showed that the cells departing the allograft had been replaced by similar recipient cells. This demonstrated that systemic and kidney graft chimerism had been established (Starzl, Demetris, Trucco et al., 1993).

Chimerism in Liver Transplantation. The chimeric nature of the liver after transplantation was first shown in 1969 in long-term survivors of orthotopic hepatic allografts. Karyotyping studies showed that when cadaveric liver grafts were obtained from opposite sex donors, the hepatocytes and endothelia of major blood vessels retained their donor specificity, whereas the entire macrophage system, including Kupffer cells, was replaced with recipient cells (Starzl, Demetris, Murase et al., 1992). It was not clear where the cells that had left the liver had gone, but their presence was confirmed in the recipient blood by detection of new donor-specific immunoglobulin types and red blood cell alloantibodies (Starzl, Demetris, Murase et al., 1992). In 1991, Dr. Robin Fox, editor of the *Lancet*, asked the authors of an article showing the chimeric nature of transplanted human intestine, ". . . if they could consider adding a few words about the fate of the donor lymphocytes?" (Starzl, Demetris, Trucco et al., 1993). This single request began an intense reexamination of data from much earlier investigations of kidney and liver transplant recipients.

For many years, the chimeric structure of the transplanted liver was thought to be unique to this organ, due to its high level of lymphoid and dendritic cells. The fate of the donor leukocyte cells was commonly assumed to have been a fate of destruction upon leaving their donor home. Later, the new residence of these cells would be found to be systemic in the recipient. Direct evidence of systemic chimerism was found in 1992 when a group of transplant surgeons and pathologists from the Pittsburgh Transplant Institute reported a state of balanced lymphodendritic cell chimerism between the host and donor liver graft. In examining eight female recipients of male donor livers with good graft function 10 to 19 years post-transplantation, evidence of the Y chromosome was found in the blood (6/8), skin (8/8), and lymph nodes (7/8). A ninth patient who required retransplantation 12 years later due to recurrent chronic viral hepatitis had chimerism in her lymph nodes, skin, jejunum, and aorta at the time of surgery (Starzl, Demetris, Trucco et al., 1992).

Chimerism in Intestinal Transplantation. The transplanted liver seems to assume a privileged tolerogenicity, which is thought to be due to its large population of migratory cells that have the ability to "seed" systemically in the recipient. This assumption of uniqueness was dispelled in 1991 when it was demonstrated first in rat models and then in human beings that all successfully transplanted intestines were indeed chimeric. Having increased the sophistication for which chimerism can be detected through cell phenotyping, differentiating donor and recipient cells has led to many more discoveries. In the intestinal transplant studies being done at the Pittsburgh Transplant Institute, it was demonstrated that the epithelium of the bowel remained that of the donor; but the lymphoid, dendritic, and other leukocytes of recipients became the dominant cells in the lamina propria, Peyer's patches, and mesenteric nodes of the donor graft (Iwaki et al., 1991). Due to the lymphoid nature of the intestine, chimerism was made easier to demonstrate. This finding caused speculation that graft chimerism might be a generic feature of all accepted grafts. In 1992, it would be demonstrated that kidneys and thoracic organs, thought to be "nonlymphoid," were also capable of both systemic and graft chimerism.

Chimerism in Thoracic Organ Transplantation. The same cell migration process occurs in the transplantation of heart and lungs. The thoracic viscera participate in this migratory process, but there does exist a quantitative difference. The liver contains the highest number of dendritic leukocytes and other potentially migratory cells, whereas the kidney and heart contain the lowest number (see Figure 5.1). When rat hearts and lungs were transplanted and not treated with immunosuppression, the heart was less

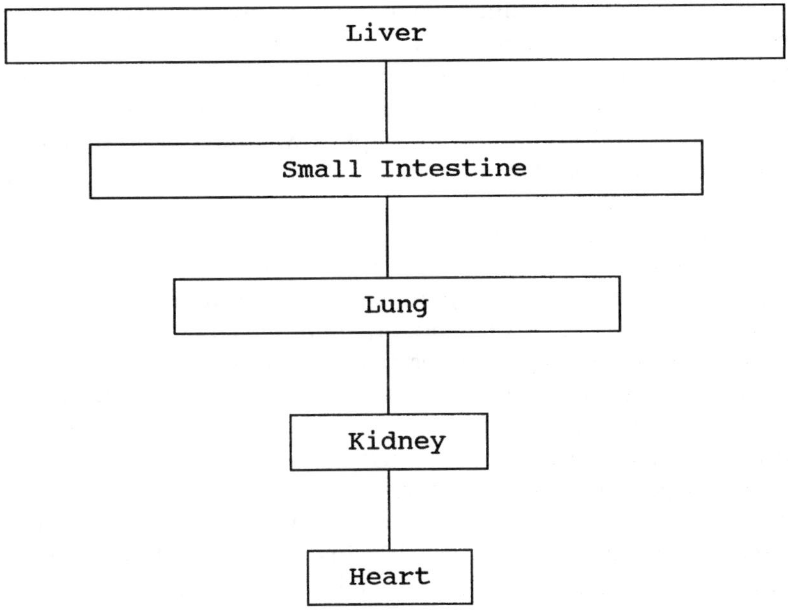

FIGURE 5.1 Hierarchy of volume of lymphoid cells by organ.

vigorously rejected than the lung. This was thought to be due to the heart being leukocyte-poor and the lung containing rich bronchus-associated lymphoid tissue. Permanent acceptance of the lung, but never the heart, has occurred after one or two doses of cyclosporine. This study concluded that this was due to the greater volume of the lung's lymphoid system, which allowed more dendritic cell migration. In September 1992, researchers at the Pittsburgh Transplant Institute obtained a biopsy of the sigmoid colon of a female patient who had received both lungs from a male donor three months earlier. The male cells in the colon showed clearly that chimerism had occurred and that the presence of these cells was not diagnostic of GVHD (Starzl, Demetris, Trucco et al., 1993).

Step Three: Augmentation of Chimerism

Chimerism appears to be the common factor in long-term transplant recipients who have successfully discontinued immunosuppression. Chimeric studies performed on these recipients have demonstrated that chimerism is present both systemically and in the donor graft and that tolerance has been achieved (Starzl et al., 1993). Why all patients do not achieve this tolerant state is still under investigation. It must be stressed, however, that achieving chimerism does not imply that true tolerance has been achieved. It may be merely a "step along the way" to developing graft tolerance/acceptance. Where in the past drug therapies to control rejection were focused on preventing two-way cellular migration and ultimately chimerism, the objective perhaps now should be to promote and even augment cellular migration while at the same time preventing graft rejection and GVHD.

If chimerism is the common factor, how can it be created or "augmented"? The answer may be through augmenting the process of cellular migration. Two-way cellular migration occurs naturally within a few minutes of revascularization of solid organ transplants. Augmenting the process involves infusing perioperatively bone marrow from the donor that contains the dendritic and leukocyte cells thought necessary to achieve a chimeric state. At the time of organ procurement, donor thoracolumbar vertebra (rich in bone marrow) is excised, prepared, filtered, and infused perioperatively after revascularization of the whole organ graft (Fontes et al., 1994). The Pittsburgh Transplant Institute has recently published a very detailed report achieving donor-cell chimerism in kidney, liver, heart, and pancreas islet transplantation using donor bone marrow infusions (Fontes et al., 1994). The next step in this research will be testing for "tolerance" or "donor-specific unresponsiveness" as evidenced through the withdrawal of immunosuppression.

Many considerations regarding chimerism and bone marrow transplant are being evaluated. Particular concerns include the following:

- The number of bone marrow infusions necessary
- The timing of the bone marrow infusion
- The amount and type of immunosuppression required post-transplant

Results will most likely show the continued need for a very individualized approach to the amount of immunosuppression, if any, required for these patients. These and many other studies currently being conducted in transplant centers across the world are allowing for transplant specialists to take the opportunity to reexamine former transplant theories and therapies.

Step Four: Patient Education Regarding Chimerism

Ideally, besides routine self-care and assessment, the recipient in a chimerism study needs to understand two concepts: the protocols of the chimerism study and the early signs of graft-versus-host disease.

Protocols for withdrawing immunosuppression and allowing the chimeric state to control graft take must be explained fully to the recipient who opts for this therapy. Recipients usually sign an investigational consent form for their individualized treatment plans. Points to be discussed should include the following:

- Expectations and limitations of the study
- Criteria for entry into the study
- Criteria for discontinuation of the study

Emphasis is placed on the fact that not all patients demonstrate the same degree of chimerism and the patient must deal with whatever degree of success is achieved.

Patient teaching should focus on the patient's potential to develop GVHD when undergoing this type of transplant technique. Although GVHD is a rare occurrence in solid organ transplantation, there is increased risk in developing GVHD with this technique of organ transplantation and the additional infusion of donor bone marrow. The first sign and symptom of GVHD presents as a dermatitis, most often as a palmar rash or a rash on top of the ears. Suspicious rashes must not be inadvertently assumed to be a rash due to drug reaction or allergies and must be reported promptly to the transplant team.

CHIMERISM AND THE FUTURE

The concept of chimerism can be applied in all areas of transplantation when researchers fully understand the process. One area of investigation is the current bone marrow protocol concerning HLA matching. It has been demonstrated that HLA mismatched donor bone marrow/solid organ transplantation can be successful without preconditioning of the recipient. One of the most controversial areas of transplantation in which chimerism has future applications is in xenotransplantation. Promoting two-way cell migration and controlling antibody development in xenotransplantation are secrets of chimerism awaiting further research.

REFERENCES

Fontes, P., Rao, A. S., Demetris, A. J., Zeevi, A., Trucco, M., Carroll, P., Rybka, W., Rudert, W. A., Ricordi, C., Dodson, F., Shapiro, R., Tzakis, A., Todo, S., Abu-Elmagd, K., Jordan, M., Fung, J. J., & Starzl, T. E. (1994). Bone marrow augmentation of donor-cell chimerism in kidney, liver, heart, and pancreas islet transplantation. *Lancet, 344,* 151–155.

Iwaki, Y., Starzl, T. E., Yagihashi, A., Taniwaki, S., Abu-Elmagd, K., Tzakis, A., Fung, J., & Todo, S. (1991). Replacement of donor lymphoid tissue in human small bowel transplants under FK506 immunosuppression. *Lancet, 337,* 818–819.

Starzl, T. E., Demetris, A. J., Murase, N., Ildstad, S., Ricordi, C., & Trucco, M. (1992). Cell migration, chimerism, and graft acceptance. *Lancet, 339,* 1579–1582.

Starzl, T. E., Demetris, A. J., Trucco, M., Murase, N., Ricordi, C., Ildstad, S., Ramos, H., Todo, S., Tzakis, A., Fung, J. J., Nalesnik, M., Zeevi, A., Rudert, W. A., & Kocova, M. (1993). Cell migration and chimerism after whole-organ transplantation: the basis of graft acceptance. *Hepatology, 17,* 1127–1152.

Starzl, T. E., Demetris, A. J., Trucco, M., Ramos, H., Zeevi, A., Rudent, W. A., Kocova, M., Ricordi, C., Ildstad, S., & Murase, N. (1992). Systemic chimerism in human female recipients of male livers. *Lancet, 340,* 876–877.

Starzl, T. E., Murase, N., Demetris, A. J., Giorda, R., Valdivia, L., & Trucco, M. (1993). Drug development and testing in relation to cell migration and chimerism. *Transplantation Proceedings, 25,* 469–472.

Steinman, R. M. (1991). The dendritic cell system and its role in immunogenicity. *Annual Review of Immunology, 9,* 271–296.

6

NEW IMMUNOSUPPRESSIVE MOLECULES FOR CONTROL OF ORGAN TRANSPLANT REJECTION

Randall E. Morris, M.D.

We are at the beginning of a revolution in the discovery, development, and application of new drugs for the control of graft rejection. This revolution is being driven by the success of the so-called xenobiotic immunosuppressants; these are small molecular-weight drugs that are produced by microorganisms or by organic synthesis. The number of these new drugs that have advanced to clinical use in just the last 5 years is more than double the number of xenobiotic immunosuppressants that have been approved for use for transplantation in the last 35 years. In addition, many of these new drugs suppress the immune system by novel mechanisms of action. These new compounds have generated a momentum that will sustain new developments in immunosuppression for many years to come.

Even if not all of the current new xenobiotic immunosuppressants are approved and widely adopted for clinical use, information gained from the study of these compounds will be the foundation for further immunosuppressive drug development. For example, when the specific benefits and limitations of the xenobiotics now in clinical trials become more clearly defined, strategies for improving these drugs and for developing different agents will come into clearer focus. In addition to the value of the study of these drugs in vitro, these compounds have proven to be essential to the understanding of fundamental immunological processes. Since these drugs block different steps leading to immune cell activation, these agents have been wielded creatively as molecular tools to discover and dissect new biochemical pathways that are critical to the immune cell response. Information from these studies is being used to draw blueprints of the immune system's circuitry that will be harnessed to design even more effective, specific, and safe means of controlling the immune response.

Although the new xenobiotic immunosuppressants are far from ideal, they represent important advances that are the result of intense research on immune suppression over nearly a decade. The field of immunosuppression is changing so rapidly that this chapter should be viewed as a snapshot of this discipline in mid-flight in late 1994. No other chapter in this book is as likely to become obsolete as rapidly as this one. For this reason, the goal of this chapter will be to introduce the reader to the new drugs that are now in clinical trials and that have the potential to be used in recipients of transplanted grafts. This introduction will endeavor to provide a logical framework that can be referred to as new information about these agents becomes available. Concepts of each drug's mechanisms of action, rather than precise details, will be provided because this area is being actively investigated and a specific account of our current beliefs would imply a level of confidence that does not truly exist. Similarly, the results of clinical trials will not be discussed in detail because most of the clinical data are from uncontrolled studies. Because the field of immunosuppression is so dynamic, this chapter should be read in conjunction with the most up-to-date articles and reviews devoted to these drugs' mechanisms of action and clinical trial result. (See Reference list.)

CATEGORIES OF NEW XENOBIOTIC IMMUNOSUPPRESSANTS

In the past, new immunosuppressants were introduced infrequently enough for those in the field to become familiar with each agent before the next new drug appeared. For example, from approximately 1960 to the mid–1980s, only three new xenobiotic drugs were widely adopted for use in transplantation: steroids, azathioprine, and cyclosporine (CsA). Poly- and monoclonal anti-T cell antibodies were also introduced during that time. In the last 12 years, nine new xenobiotics have entered clinical trials, and eight of these began testing in the last 5 years alone. This explosion of new agents is a considerable challenge to those who realize that to understand the future of transplantation, one must understand the differences and similarities among these new drugs. The rate of progress is now so rapid that instead of assimilating information about one new drug every few years, several drugs must be understood simultaneously. To minimize confusion, these drugs can be categorized by structure, origin, and mechanisms of action. These categories provide an outline that enables the drugs to be grouped in ways that compare their similarities and contrast their differences.

The structures of CsA and several of the new xenobiotic immunosuppressants are shown in Figure 6.1. Two of the new agents, cyclosporin G (CsG) and IMM 125 are structurally related analogues of CsA and are not shown. The structures of the other seven new drugs are shown. Only two of these seven drugs bear some structural resemblance to each other: FK506 (tacrolimus) and rapamycin (RPM, sirolimus). The remaining five drugs are leflunomide (LFM), mizoribine (MZR), mycophenolate mofetil (MMF), brequinar sodium (BQR), and deoxyspergualin (DSG). None of these five compounds is structurally related to each other or to the other four new agents. It is important to understand that the structures shown in Figure 6.1 are the structures of the drugs in the forms in which they are administered. LFM, MZR, and MMF are prodrugs and undergo a change in structure to become the active form of the drug. Before MMF was produced, the active form of the drug, mycophenolic acid (MPA), was administered. Therefore, MMF and MPA will be referred to interchangeably in this chapter.

Categorizing the nine new xenobiotics by origin is relatively simple. For example, the CsA analogue, CsG, as well as FK506, RPM, and MZR are the metabolic products of bacteria or fungi. BQR and LFM are produced by total organic synthesis. The other CsA analogue, IMM 125, as well as MMF and DSG are fermentation products that have been modified chemically after their isolation. Therefore, the origins of these new agents fall into the following categories: natural product, synthetic, or semisynthetic.

Most important of all is the categorization of these new drugs by their mechanisms of immunosuppressive action. This is shown in Figure 6.2. Despite the similarities and differences among these drugs' structures and origins, there is no clear relationship between these categories and the drugs' mechanisms of action. CsA and its analogues are structurally distinct from FK506; but CsA, its analogues, and FK506 suppress immune

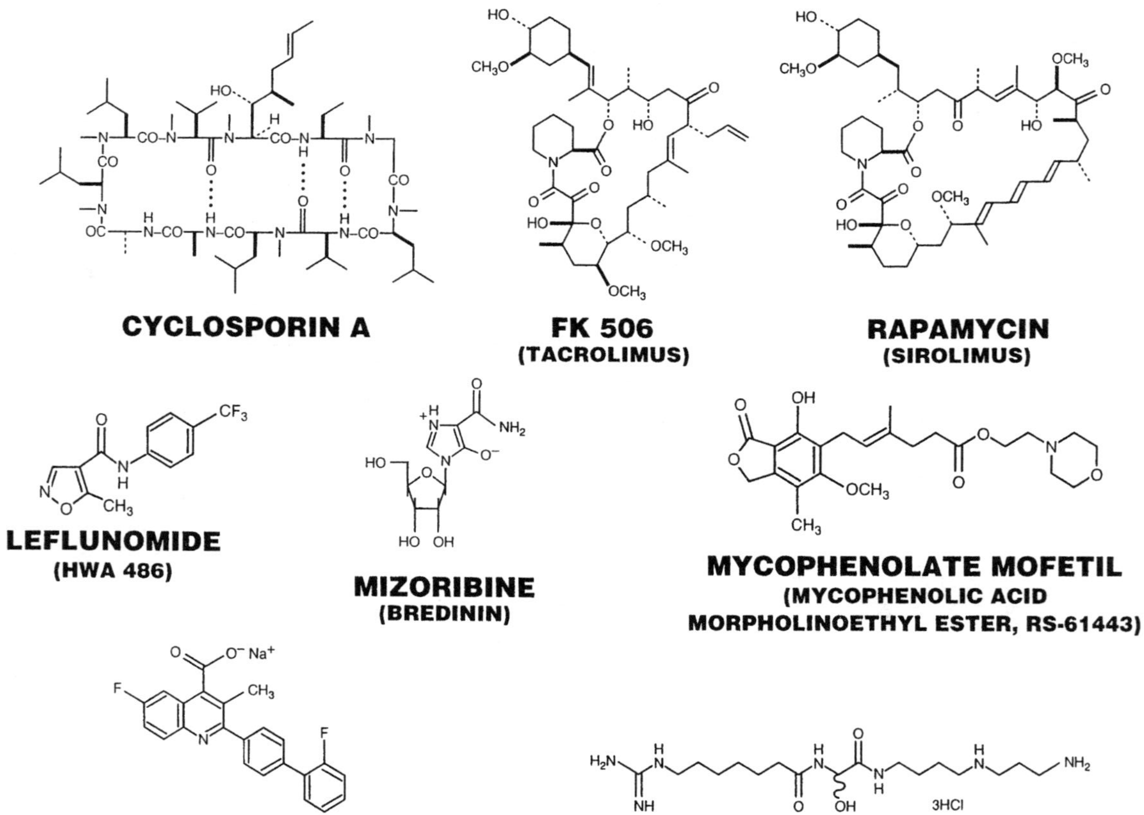

FIGURE 6.1 Structures of new immunosuppressive drugs.

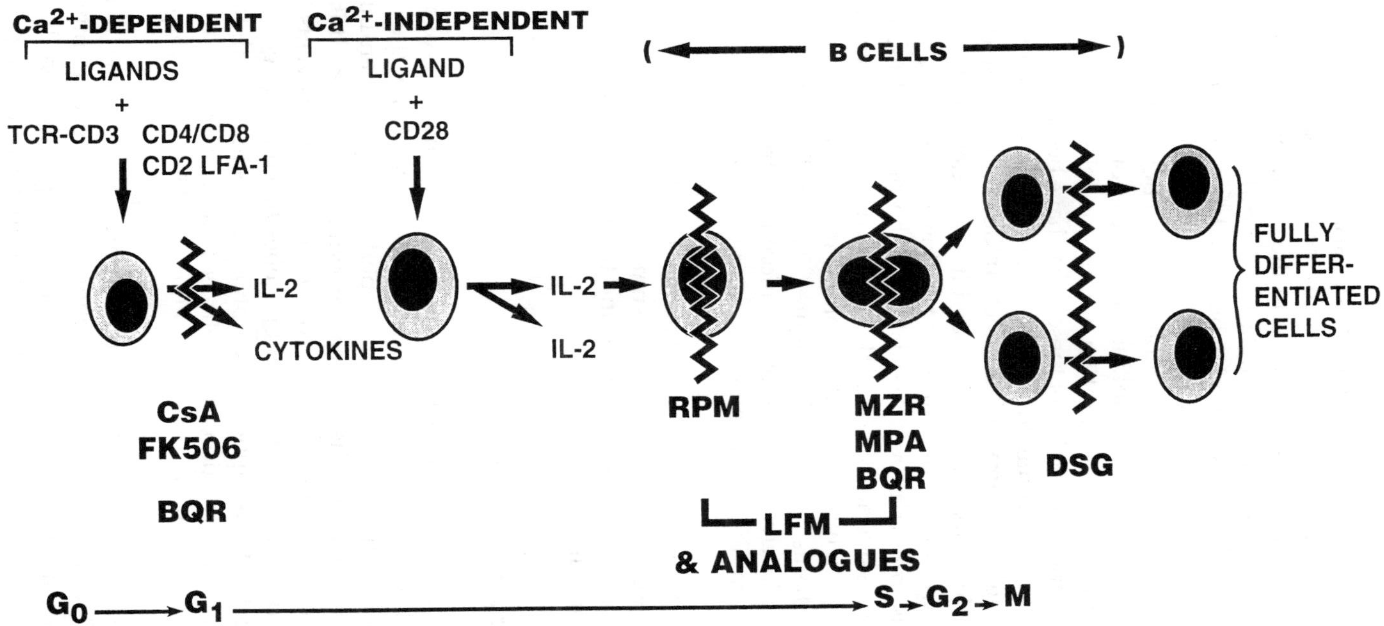

FIGURE 6.2 Possible sites of action in T cells of new xenobiotic immunosuppressants.

cell function by inhibiting cytokine synthesis. RPM is structurally similar to FK506, yet RPM does not block cytokine synthesis. RPM is a natural product that is structurally dissimilar to the synthetically produced LFM, yet both block the action of growth factors by different mechanisms. MZR and MPA are structurally dissimilar, but both block purine synthesis. BQR is the only drug that blocks pyrimidine synthesis, except for LFM, which may also have a mechanism of action similar to BQR. DSG does not inhibit the synthesis or action of cytokines and does not block DNA synthesis, but it does suppress the maturation of immune cells.

As the mechanisms of action of these drugs have begun to be more clearly understood, it has become possible to reconcile the apparent incongruity between a drug's structure and its effect on the immune system. Structure-function relationships will be discussed in more detail below. Regardless of how well we now understand the relationship between structure and function, it is important to appreciate that the proposed mechanisms of immunosuppressive action for all these new drugs are derived from studies done completely in vitro. Therefore, it remains to be shown that the proposed mechanisms outlined in Figure 6.2 faithfully represent the actions of these drugs in vivo. Furthermore, as more is learned about these drugs, other mechanisms of immunosuppressive action are likely to be discovered.

The remainder of this chapter will discuss each drug as part of the category that describes its mechanism of action. Recently, detailed information on each of these new agents has been summarized in reviews or proceedings of conferences. These references and these articles should be referred to for additional information.

Cytokine Synthesis Inhibitors

Three of the newest immunosuppressants have mechanisms of action that mimic CsA. It is now known that CsA binds to proteins in the cytoplasm known as cyclophilins. The drug-cyclophilin complex then inhibits the enzymatic activity of another protein known as calcineurin. It is believed that calcineurin plays an important role in the cascade of events that leads to the transcription of certain cytokine genes (such as the gene for IL-2). By inhibiting the transcription of lymphocyte-specific growth factors, the proliferation and activation of T cells is halted. Although CsA cannot directly inhibit B cell activation, T cell-dependent B cell responses are inhibited.

CsA is close to the ideal immunosuppressant because it does not depend on T cell depletion for its actions and because its immunosuppressive effects are restricted to T cells undergoing activation. The primary drawbacks to the use of CsA are the nephrotoxicity, diabetogenesis, and hypertension associated with its administration. It now appears that the toxic effects of CsA are mediated by complexes between CsA, cyclophilin, and calcineurin—the same complexes that are responsible for this drug's immunosuppressive actions. As a result, it has been difficult to create analogues of CsA that retain immunosuppressive efficacy and are also less toxic. Recently, two new analogues, CsG and IMM 125, have begun to be evaluated in the clinic. CsG appears to have a greater therapeutic index than its parent (it is less nephrotoxic), but the hepatotoxicity of IMM 125 has caused clinical trials in transplantation to be abandoned. So much effort has been expended in the search for analogues with greater therapeutic indexes that this research effort is reaching the point of diminishing returns. Because the initial steps in the pathways leading to suppression of T cell proliferation and to toxicity appear to be identical, and because CsA and its analogues block these steps, there is little opportunity to design molecules that are immunosuppressive and not at all toxic.

The third drug that mediates its immunosuppressive effects by interfering with the transcription of cytokine genes is FK506. FK506 also inhibits the activity of calcineurin after the drug has complexed with its cytoplasmic-binding protein, FKBP. Since FK506 binds to FKBP much more avidly than CsA binds to cyclophilin, FK506 is a more potent immunosuppressant. In certain instances, FK506 has been able to reverse rejection that has been resistant to conventional immunosuppression. Although the greatest experience with FK506 has been in liver allograft recipients, this drug has also been evaluated in renal and heart transplant patients. FK506 has been used to prevent and to treat liver and heart graft rejection with good results. It is less clear whether this drug offers a significant improvement over CsA in kidney graft recipients. The use of FK506 appears to have several advantages. First, the need for conventional immunosuppressants (monoclonal anti-T cell antibodies, azathioprine, and steroids) has been reduced. Second, FK506 can be used to treat rejection simply by increasing the dose.

As expected from its mechanism of action, the toxicity profile of FK506 is similar to CsA. FK506 is nephrotoxic, and blood levels must be kept within narrow limits to ensure that nephrotoxicity is minimized. It is unlikely that analogues of FK506 will offer vastly superior therapeutic indexes because the mechanisms of immunosuppressive action of FK506 appear to be inseparable from the biochemical pathways that cause toxicity.

Inhibitors of Cytokine Action

There are two drugs that define this new class of immunosuppressants: RPM and LFM. Neither inhibits the synthesis of cytokines, but both block the actions of immune as well as nonimmune cytokines and growth factors. Although both RPM and LFM appear to affect cells similarly at a superficial level, the precise mechanisms by which they mediate their effects are different. Unlike CsA and its analogues and FK506, RPM and LFM also act directly on B cells to inhibit their functions.

RPM is structurally similar to FK506 and must bind to FKBPs to be immunosuppressive. Since the RPM-FKBP complex does not interact with calcineurin, the toxicity profile of RPM differs from CsA and FK506. Preclinical animal toxicology indicates that RPM is not as nephrotoxic as FK506. The exact biochemical events responsible for the inhibition of cytokine and growth factor action by the RPM-FKBP complex are far from clear, but the pharmacological target of the complex now appears to be a lipid kinase. T cells can be stimulated to proliferate by pathways (calcium-independent signaling, see Figure 6.2) that bypass the T cell receptor, and their pathways are not blocked by CsA or FK506. Stimulation of T cell proliferation via the CD28 pathway or by the interaction of IL-2 with its receptor are blocked by RPM.

It is clear that RPM is an unusually potent drug for the prevention and treatment of allograft rejection in experimental animals. Its ability to prevent graft vascular disease in rat heart allografts may be due to a combination of its suppressive effects on T and B cells and its ability to block the effects of growth factors that stimulate the proliferation of intimal smooth muscle cells. The ultimate importance of this drug will have to await the outcome of clinical trials that are now under way. Phase I studies are being conducted to determine the maximum tolerated dose of this drug and its dose-limiting side effects. These data plus information from Phase II efficacy studies in transplant patients will determine the therapeutic index of this agent.

LFM is a prodrug that is converted almost immediately after administration to the active form of the drug. The current speculation regarding the mechanism of action of LFM is that it blocks the activity of selected tyrosine kinases associated with cell surface growth factor receptors. As a result, the normal transduction of signals after the interaction of a growth factor with its receptor is blocked. There are data that also suggest that this drug inhibits growth factor action by blocking pyrimidine synthesis. LFM has been studied most thoroughly in patients with rheumatoid arthritis and has been quite effective for the treatment of advanced forms of this condition. The analysis of safety data from this study is incomplete, but so far it does not appear that LFM has any substantial toxic effects on specific organ systems. Information on the immunosuppressive efficacy of LF in animal transplant recipients is limited, but the data show that it very effectively prolongs the survival of kidney, skin, and heart grafts in rodents. Recent studies have shown it to be an effective agent for the suppression of acute rejection in nonhuman and dog organ allograft recipients when combined with CsA.

In preclinical transplant animal models, both RPM and LFM have been shown to be highly effective when combined with CsA. It is likely that this type of combination therapy could be useful in the clinic because it may allow the doses of CsA to be reduced to levels that are non-nephrotoxic. The use of drugs that block distinct steps in the immune response and that have nonoverlapping toxicity is a rational means of improving immunosuppression while at the same time reducing systemic toxicity.

Inhibitors of DNA Synthesis

There are three drugs in this category: MZR, MPA (or its prodrug form MM), and BQR (and perhaps LFM, see above). Each of these is a potential alternative to azathioprine. There is one important theoretical advantage that both MZR and MPA have over azathioprine. T cells and B cells rely, more than other cells, on the de novo pathway for the synthesis of purine nucleotides. Unlike other cells, T cells and B cells cannot use the salvage pathway for purine biosynthesis. MZR and MPA are relatively selective inhibitors of T cell and B cell DNA synthesis because both these drugs block the activity of a single critical enzyme responsible for the synthesis of purines in the de novo pathway. In contrast, azathioprine blocks many enzymes that are required for DNA synthesis, and is a less specific inhibitor of immune cell proliferation than either MZR or MPA.

MZR has been used as an alternative for azathioprine for about a dozen years in transplant recipients in Japan. In those studies, less myelotoxicity was noted in patients on MZR compared to azathioprine. More extensive studies in transplantation have been done with MPA. Preclinical work has shown that this compound prolongs the survival of organ allografts in rodents and large animals. It has also been found to be effective for the reversal of ongoing rejection in these models. Most of the clinical studies have concentrated on the effects of MMF in renal transplant patients. These Phase II trials have shown that there is a relationship between the dose and the incidence of graft rejection. Other studies showed that MMF is able to reverse rejection in patients that were refractory to treatment with conventional immunosuppressants. MMF has been used in rodent transplant models to prevent graft vascular disease, and this application may also be relevant to its use in patients.

BQR does not directly inhibit purine synthesis but does block the action of a key enzyme in the pathway leading to pyrimidine synthesis. Although BQR failed as an anticancer agent, its use in patients with malignant diseases provided information on its safety and pharmacokinetics. Since high doses of BQR and continued use have been shown to be myelotoxic, the rationale for its use as an immunosuppressant depends on the assumption that immune cells are more sensitive to its antimetabolic effects than nonimmune cells. This assumption has been borne out in studies of the immunosuppressive efficacy of BQR in rodent graft recipients. These experiments have shown that BQR is able to prevent rejection and very effectively halts ongoing rejection. It has also been used effectively for the prolongation of hamster-to-rat xenografts. Experiments that are currently ongoing will determine the efficacy of this drug in large animal recipients of organ allografts. Since BQR has been shown to produce immunosuppression in rodent allograft recipients that is at least additive when combined with CsA, it is likely that BQR will be used as adjunctive therapy in patients. This drug is in Phase II trials in renal transplant recipients.

Inhibitor of Cell Maturation

DSG not only has a structure that differs from all the other new xenobiotic immunosuppressants, it also suppresses the immune system by means that are distinct from other agents. For example, in vitro studies have shown that DSG is not an effective inhibitor of cytokine synthesis, the actions of cytokines, or DNA synthesis. Despite its apparent inability to suppress these steps in immune activation that are the target of other drugs, DSG is an effective immunosuppressant. Its true mechanism of immunosuppressive action is unknown, but by a process of elimination, it appears that DSG blocks the immune response by halting the maturation of T and B cells into fully functional effector cells. This drug, like RPM, LFM, and the antimetabolites, directly suppresses T cells and B cells in vitro.

In vivo, DSG has been used to prevent rejection of rodent allo- and xenografts. In nonhuman primates treated with a short course of DSG plus long-term therapy with CsA, prolonged graft survival was seen. DSG has also been found to halt advanced rejection in rodent and large-animal graft recipients. This activity prompted the first clinical trials in Japan in renal allograft recipients. These patients had continued to reject despite a variety of conventional immunosuppressive treatments. Although the trials were not controlled, the results appeared to support the belief that this drug was effective for this application. Clinical trials are now being conducted in the United States in high-risk renal allograft recipients who have previously rejected one or more grafts within a year of transplantation. DSG can now only be administered intravenously, so these patients are receiving a short induction course in conjunction with conventional immunosuppressants. If the results of this trial indicate that

DSG is effective, a more extensive and controlled Phase II trial will be undertaken.

SUMMARY

The proliferation of new xenobiotic drugs offers the potential to benefit transplantation in many ways. In theory, the use of drugs with different mechanisms of action and nonoverlapping toxicities should increase the overall immunosuppressive efficacy without increasing systemic toxicity. The variety of new drugs will enable this assumption to be tested in the clinic. Already these new molecules have been used to uncover new knowledge of how immune cells respond to activation. This understanding, in turn, will be the foundation for the discovery and development of a new generation of immunosuppressants. In the meantime, the current drugs need to be studied much more thoroughly in vitro, in animal transplant models, and in clinical trials so that they can be used intelligently and to their maximum advantage. We now have more drugs than ever before that directly suppress B cell function, and these drugs may be especially valuable for xenograft recipients.

Compared to the situation over the last 30 years, the present number and variety of new immunosuppressants is very great. It is important to remember, however, that the immune system is exceedingly complex. Therefore, in the future, the number of new drugs of all types will continue to increase. As the complexity of immunosuppression increases, a greater premium will be placed on drugs that are clearly safer and more effective than the drugs that now exist. This competitive environment will ensure that continued progress is made.

REFERENCES

Annual American Society of Transplant Surgeons postgraduate course: Advances in immunosuppression. (1991). *Clinical Transplantation, 5,* 475–599 (part 2).

Bartlett, R. R., Dimitrijevic, M., Mattar, T., Ziclinski, T., Germann, T., Rüde, E., Thoenes, G. H., Küchle, C. C. A., Schorlemmer, H.-U., Bremer, E., Finnegan, A., & Schleyerbach, R. (1992). Leflunomide (HWA 486): A novel immunomodulating compound for the treatment of autoimmune disorders and reactions leading to transplant rejection. *Agents and Actions, 32,* 10–21.

Cramer, D. V., Chapman, F. A., Jaffee, B. D., Jones, E. A., Knoop, M., Hreha-Eiras, G., & Makowka, L. (1992). The effect of a new immunosuppressive drug, brequinar sodium, on heart, liver, and kidney allograft rejection in the rat. *Transplantation, 53,* 303–308.

Dayton, J. S., Turka, L. A., Thompson, C. B., & Mitchell, B. S. (1992). Comparison of the effects of mizoribine with those of azathioprine, 6-mercaptopurine and mycophenolic acid on T lymphocyte proliferation and purine ribonucleotide metabolism. *Molecular Pharmaceuticals, 41,* 671–676.

Morris, R. E. (1992a). Immunopharmacology of new xenobiotic immunosuppressive molecules. *Seminars in Nephrology, 12,* 304–314.

Morris, R. E. (1992b). Rapamycins: Antifungal, antitumor and immunosuppressive macrolides. *Transplantation Reviews, 6,* 39–87.

Morris, R. E. (1993). Overview of immunosuppressive drugs for transplantation: Where are we? How did we get here? and Where are we going? *Clinical Transplantation, 7,* 138–145 (Part 2).

Proceedings of the First International Congress on FK 506. (1991). *Transplantation Proceedings, 23,* 2709–3380.

Sigal, N. H., & Dumont, F. J. (1992). Cyclosporin A, FK-506 and rapamycin: Pharmacological probes of lymphocyte signal transduction. *Annual Review of Immunology, 10,* 519–560.

Thomson, A. W. (Ed.). (1992). *The molecular biology of immunosuppression.* New York: John Wiley and Sons.

Transplant Proceedings: Ten years of cyclosporine in clinical practice: Past, present and future in transplantation immunology (1992). *Transplantation Proceedings, 25,* 1–99.

PART III

Women's Issues in Transplantation

7

EFFECTS OF TRANSPLANTATION ON THE FEMALE REPRODUCTIVE SYSTEM

Jacqueline Lever, R.N., M.S.N.

Organ transplantation is an accepted therapeutic option for end-stage liver and renal disease. End-stage renal disease and end-stage liver disease often lead to years of amenorrhea and subsequent infertility in women. Following transplantation and the resumption of normal menses, these women become fertile and are faced with choices concerning pregnancy or birth control. Little has been written on these women's health issues in the field of transplantation. This chapter will address a few of these issues.

AMENORRHEA IN END-STAGE DISEASES

Changes in the menstrual patterns as well as loss of libido, atrophy of the breasts, and decreased growth of body hair, especially axillary hair, in patients with liver disease were reported by two sources, Lloyd and Bearn (Bearn, Kunkel, & Slater, 1956; Lloyd & Williams, 1948). Amenorrhea is also recognized as a complication of all types of end-stage or chronic liver disease, although the incidence is higher in patients with cirrhosis and advanced hepatocellular failure than in patients with biliary disease and predominant cholestasis. Women suffering from chronic renal failure or end-stage renal disease also usually demonstrate loss of libido, anovulatory bleeding, or amenorrhea (Lau & Scott, 1985; Penn, Makowski, & Harris, 1980). It is interesting that amenorrhea usually develops early in the course of various end-stage diseases, and it is that single presenting symptom that finally motivates the patient to see her primary care provider, whether it be her family physician or the gynecologist. Some physicians miss this very significant symptom, recognizing those that occur later such as oliguria, ascites, and/or jaundice as being much more serious. At least 48% of those women diagnosed with end-stage liver disease and who are in their reproductive years have amenorrhea. In addition, excessive intake of ethanol increases the frequency of menstrual disturbances, miscarriages, and abortions. Current literature (Becker, 1993; Cundy, O'Grady, & Williams, 1990) still does not provide complete clarification of this phenomenon. Either the information is seen as insufficient, or the observations are thought to be linked to hypothalamic-pituitary dysfunction.

Pregnancy can and does, although rarely, occur in patients with end-stage kidney disease or postnecrotic cirrhosis, chronic active hepatitis, or biliary cirrhosis. Pregnancy is very uncommon in patients with Laennec's cirrhosis. Spontaneous abortion presents a significant risk to those cirrhotic women without a shunt. It is common to see early termination of the pregnancy in patients with end-stage kidney and liver disease (Cheng, 1977).

TRANSPLANTATION AND MENSTRUATION

During the past two decades, women with end-stage renal or liver disease have elected to undergo solid organ transplantation with increasing frequency. As their lives return to some normalcy, ovulation reoccurs and menstruation resumes. Amenorrhea can disappear as early as 1 month after transplantation in certain patients. Normally in patients receiving kidney transplantation, the mean time for menses to reappear is 6 months. Normal menstrual cycle is reestablished usually within 10 months in patients receiving a liver transplant. As a result, pregnancy occurs frequently among those women who have received a kidney or liver transplant. Pregnancy is also seen in women who have had heart, heart/lung, and pancreas transplants, but in significantly smaller numbers.

TRANSPLANTATION AND PREGNANCY

Kidney Transplant Patients

Following a successful kidney transplantation, there is a significant improvement in the quality of life of a patient. These patients often return to normal working life and make significant contributions to society. With an increased number of patients being able to conceive, there has been a steady increase in the number of pregnancies in kidney transplant patients.

The first documented case of a successful pregnancy after transplantation was reported by Murray, Reid, Harrison, and Merrill in 1963. The mother had received a kidney from her twin sister and had two successful pregnancies, the first a little over a year following the transplantation and the second two years later. The next few reported successful pregnancies were in patients who had received a living-related donor kidney. The first pregnancy occurring in a patient who had received a cadaveric kidney transplant was reported by Caplan, Dossetor, and Maughan in 1970. The patient suffered from chronic bilateral pyelonephritis and hydronephrosis and had experienced two miscarriages prior to transplantation, at 6 months and 31½ weeks of gestation. Six months after cadaveric kidney transplant, she conceived and 35$\frac{5}{7}$ weeks later spontaneously delivered an infant weighing 1955 gm (21% underweight for gestation). During her pregnancy, she was maintained on prednisone and received irradiation to her kidney. Along with other complications, including rejection at 33 weeks, her chest film showed a fungus ball that was diagnosed as *Aspergillus fumigates,* and she showed *Candida albicans* in her sputum. After a successful delivery, she never returned to good health and died just a little more than a year later of left ventricular hypertrophy, pericardial effusion, and chronic rejection. The child continued to develop normally both physically and immunologically.

In the 1970s and 1980s, Israel Penn reported his observations on both living related and cadaveric kidney transplant patients who had conceived subsequent to the transplantation (Penn, Makowski, Droegemueller, Halgrimson, & Starzl, 1971; Penn, Makowski, & Harris, 1980). In general, those kidney patients who had problems before getting pregnant seemed to continue to have those same problems (i.e., deterioration of renal function and difficulty controlling hypertension) during their pregnancy. However, those patients who had good graft function and satisfactory control of blood pressure and who were on maintenance doses of immunosuppression seemed to have fairly normal pregnancies. In this group of patients, the incidence of preeclampsia was 27%; prematurity occurred 49% of the time; and 30% of the infants had one or more serious, sometimes fatal complications such as congenital anomalies, respiratory distress, or infection. Generally, these patients were primarily under immunosuppression with prednisone and azathioprine while a few were treated with cyclosporine and prednisone. Davison (1987) summarized the 2,309 pregnancies in 1,594 transplant patients. According to this report, at least 1 in 50 women who have had a kidney transplant become pregnant, and 90% of these pregnancies are successful. However, a 30% incidence of preeclampsia, a 30% incidence of pregnancy-induced hypertension, a 40% chance of abortion in the first trimester, and nearly 50% chance of preterm delivery continues to be of concern. It should also be noted that 20% of the newborns are small for their respective gestational ages. Since the allograft is still placed extraperitoneally in the iliac fossa, vaginal delivery is possible in the kidney transplant patient. Ultrasound would of course be indicated if the obstetrician suspected cephalopelvic disproportion.

Liver Transplant Patients

Since liver transplantation has become an accepted method of treating patients with end-stage liver disease, an increase in the number of pregnancies among this patient population has been reported. Children who had received liver transplants in the 1980s are now well into their reproductive years and face the possibility of conception. Eleven percent of female liver transplant patients are in their reproductive years (Scantlebury et al., 1990). Since the introduction of cyclosporine in 1980, the quality of life of these patients has improved, and they lead somewhat normal lifestyles. Pregnancy has become a reality for many of these patients.

The first pregnancy after liver transplantation was reported by Walcott, Derick, Jolley, Schmid, and Snyder in 1978. This patient had persistent amenorrhea after transplant, was given clomiphene citrate daily for 5 consecutive days, and finally tested positive for pregnancy approximately 40 days later. She had waited nearly 18 months after transplant to conceive. She was maintained on azathioprine and prednisone. She delivered a healthy, 2,400-gm infant by spontaneous vaginal delivery at 40½ weeks of gestation.

Current findings report that approximately 60% of the pregnancies among liver transplant patients were unplanned. The mean age of these women at the time of pregnancy was 25. The average interval from time of transplant to the diagnosis of pregnancy was 26 months, with a range of 5 months to 11 years. The mean gestational age was 34⁷⁄₁₀ weeks, with

55% of the babies being born premature and 63% requiring cesarean sections. Several cases of intrauterine growth retardation have been reported. There have been no cases of congenital abnormalities.

PROBLEMS WITH PREGNANCIES IN TRANSPLANT PATIENTS

There are significant concerns with regard to the mother in terms of the anticipated complications she may experience during pregnancy, as well as with the fetus in terms of normal development (see Table 7.1). Potential risks to the mother include graft loss, hypertension, anemia, and, in the liver transplant patient, hyperbilirubinemia. Since these mothers are maintained on such immunosuppressive agents as cyclosporine or tacrolimus, azathioprine, and perhaps prednisone, problems suffered by the mother and those that must be cautiously watched include infection, hypertension, and gastrointestinal disorders. The biggest concern during pregnancy is maintaining the graft function. In liver transplant patients, a 35% incidence of increased hepatic enzymes has been reported by Scantlebury et al. (1990). However, only one case of acute rejection was seen in 20 pregnancies.

Physiological changes associated with pregnancy may alter the distribution, metabolism, and clearance of drugs such as tacrolimus (Prograf) or cyclosporine. Changes in red cell count and plasma volume expansion, as well as changes in body weight and body fat content, may cause a *lowering* of cyclosporine concentrations. This does not imply that doses should be changed, but rather emphasizes the importance of therapeutic monitoring in these patients and the need for additional studies in this patient population.

TABLE 7.1 Risks Associated With Pregnancy in Transplant Patients

- Preterm delivery
- Preeclampsia
- Hypertension
- Anemia
- Abortion in first trimester
- Graft loss (minimal)
- Hyperbilirubinemia (OLTX)

TRANSPLANTATION DURING PREGNANCY

There have been several reports of transplant surgery being carried out during pregnancy (Fair, Feng, Merritt, & Burdick, 1990; Laifer, Darby, Scantlebury, Harger, & Caritis, 1990), though it should be emphasized that this is by no means recommended.

Kidney Transplant Patient

One patient was on dialysis 6 months and, unknown to her attending physician, was at 13 to 14 weeks of gestation when she received a kidney. She experienced premature onset of labor at 34 to 35 weeks and delivered a 1,870-gm infant with Apgar scores of 5 and 7. This infant was treated for mild respiratory distress syndrome. Also present were hyperbilirubinemia and hypothyroidism, as well as an atrial septal defect.

Liver Transplant Patients

Two cases of liver transplants being performed in pregnant patients, both suffering from fulminant hepatic failure and both requiring retransplant due to primary nonfunction of the graft, have been reported. In one case, postoperative recovery was complicated with the development of a severe reactivation of cytomegalovirus infection with pneumonitis and pancreatitis, which was treated with gancyclovir and reduction in the amount of immunosuppression. The infant was delivered by cesarean section, weighed 2 lb 4 oz with an Apgar score of 3 and 9, and was treated for respiratory distress and transient hyperbilirubinemia. The child improved and subsequently became well-developed. The second case was complicated by acute renal failure and a severe exacerbation of a previously unknown genital herpes infection, requiring intravenous acyclovir. Because of a sinusoidal fetal heart rate pattern, the baby was delivered by cesarean section, but the neonate died 4 days later. Autopsy revealed necrotizing enterocolitis with bowel perforation and peritonitis, hyaline membrane disease, and intracranial hemorrhage.

CARE OF THE PREGNANT TRANSPLANT PATIENT

This section is presented as a summary and general overview for the health care provider who will be caring for the pregnant transplant patient. This information comes from many recommended sources and is meant to provide guidelines in managing the care of this patient population (see Table 7.2).

The pregnant transplant patient should seek the services of an obstetrician who deals with the "high-risk" patient population and who will work well coordinating the care of this patient. Perhaps the single most important factor that must be considered when dealing with the pregnant transplant patient is the need to plan the pregnancy effectively. Counseling should begin during the transplant evaluation process, and the woman should continue to see her gynecologist while awaiting transplant. She should discuss the possibility of pregnancy with the transplant team as well. Support and guidance should be provided, and issues such as the patient's prognosis and quality of life issues, as well as consideration on the part of the patient as to whether she will live long enough to raise a child, should be addressed. After transplant, someone from the transplant team, often the nurse coordinator, should address the concerns of resuming a healthy, normal sex life. Health care workers should listen to the patient's concerns and encourage her to resume regular checkups with her gynecologist.

Ideally, in order to optimize the chances of a successful pregnancy, the patient should consider pregnancy only after the following three conditions have been met:

- Graft function is stable with no evidence of rejection.
- Any known medical conditions are under control (hypertension, diabetes).
- Immunosuppression is being administered at maintenance levels.

The literature indicates that when these conditions exist, the chance of producing a healthy infant and experiencing a somewhat normal pregnancy are much more promising. However, several factors, including persistent amenorrhea, do not always permit this situation to exist, and the patient is surprised with the results of her positive pregnancy test.

TABLE 7.2 Important Interventions When Providing Nursing Care to Pregnant Transplant Patients

- Effective counseling and planning
- Close interaction between patient and nurse coordinator
- Control of any medical condition (hypertension, diabetes)
- Maintain stable graft function
- Gynecological/obstetrical care managed by "high-risk" physician
- Choose knowledgeable pediatrician to provide care after delivery

Effective communication must exist between the patient and, ideally, the father, and all members of the health care team. This team includes the transplant surgeons, the patient care coordinators, the gynecologist/obstetrician, the pharmacist, and those who provide psychosocial as well as financial support (i.e., the insurance company). All findings should be recorded and copied to the appropriate resources. Any concerns should be reported to the appropriate caregiver before effective planning can begin.

CARE DURING PREGNANCY

Prenatal Considerations

Essential Testing. It is recommended that a complete laboratory profile be obtained at the first prenatal visit. This would include a complete blood count, including platelet count, and a chemistry panel including BUN, serum creatinine, electrolytes, and liver function studies. It should be noted that alkaline phosphatase is known to increase during normal pregnancy. It is essential to monitor the immunosuppressive agents administered. A 24-hour creatinine clearance, as well as urinalysis for microscopic evaluation, should be obtained. Glucose tolerance tests should be carried out during the first trimester and repeated at 24 to 28 weeks of gestation. CMV and HSV titers, as well as Rh screening, should be performed. The patient should be instructed to record her weight and blood pressure accurately during the pregnancy. Ultrasound should be scheduled at 16 to 20 weeks' gestation and repeated as needed during the final trimester (see Table 7.3).

Monitoring for Infection. The possible risks associated with infection must always be a prime concern on the part of the caregiver. Prophylactic antibiotics such as trimethoprim (known to cause hyperbilirubinemia in the infant), nystatin, and acyclovir should be continued. The patient should seek the guidance of a competent pharmacist who is qualified in the field of solid organ transplantation to follow the course of all prescribed medications. Cytomegalovirus infections can be life-threatening to both mother and infant. Therapeutic benefits of ganciclovir prophylaxis have not been clearly established. Strict aseptic technique is required when examining the patient as well as during the delivery process. Prophylactic antibiotics are recommended during delivery, whether it be vaginal or cesarean section.

TABLE 7.3 Monitoring of Pregnant Patients

- CMV, HSV, and Rh screening
- Strict aseptic technique during all procedures
- Complete blood profile
- 24-hour urine for creatinine clearance
- Therapeutic monitoring of immunosuppressive agents
- Ultrasound at 16 to 20 weeks (repeat as necessary)
- Glucose tolerance test (at least first trimester)
- Prophylactic antibiotics

Monitoring for Rejection. Rejection is another concern that must also be considered. Effective monitoring of kidney and liver function tests should alert the physician to any suspicion of rejection. Dosing of immunosuppressive agents, such as cyclosporine or tacrolimus, does not in general need to be increased to accommodate the weight gain and increase of blood volume associated with pregnancy. However, therapeutic monitoring of those drugs is important. Cyclosporine and tacrolimus are nephrotoxic, and cyclosporine more than tacrolimus causes hypertension. It is often difficult to distinguish between hypertension and early preeclampsia. Close monitoring of the patient is necessary. Here again, it should be emphasized that baseline (prior to pregnancy) information such as blood pressure and serum creatinine levels should be compared. Studies indicate that cyclosporine and tacrolimus are present in the cord blood, placenta, amniotic fluid, and breast milk. Neither has been proven to cause congenital abnormalities or chromosomal aberrations in animal studies, as is the case with azathioprine. Since cyclosporine and tacrolimus are excreted in breast milk, breastfeeding is contraindicated in those patients receiving these drugs because chronic effects of exposure to low doses of these agents to the newborn are not completely characterized.

Rejection can and may occur in the pregnant patient, just as frequently as a nonpregnant patient. However, often a bolus of steroids or mild increase of steroid therapy may arrest a case of rejection. Biopsies should be done if indicated. It is most important to address any patient complaints such as lethargy, decreased urinary output, fever, or tenderness over the graft.

Postpartum Considerations

A summary of suggestions for caring for the pregnant transplant patient must also include consideration of care of the patient after delivery (see Table 7.4). During the brief interval after delivery, careful therapeutic

TABLE 7.4 Postpartum Care

- Therapeutic monitoring of immunosuppressive agents
- Counseling on selection of birth control method
- Regular Pap smears and mammograms as indicated by gynecologist
- Follow-up with pediatrician

drug monitoring of immunosuppressive medication is important because of the physiological alterations of pregnancy that resolve during the postpartum period. Discussion regarding selection of an effective method of contraception must be addressed. It is not recommended that the patient consider birth control pills because of the risks associated with thromboembolism and hypertension as well as possible effects of contraceptives on the levels of immunosuppressive drugs. Intrauterine devices pose a threat of infection and uncontrolled bleeding that can lead to anemia. The use of Norplant has not been evaluated. Chemical and mechanical barriers such as creams, foams, condoms, and diaphragms are the recommended choices. The patient may want to consider a permanent method of sterilization for herself or her spouse. It is vital that she schedule regular visits to her gynecologist/obstetrician and have Pap smears and mammograms when recommended.

Care of Infant. Finally, it is also important for the mother to have made arrangements to see a pediatrician who understands the transplant process to provide care for her new infant. It is recommended that the patient see the pediatrician prior to delivery to discuss concerns and plan neonatal care (see Table 7.5). Close monitoring must be provided to monitor risk of infection in the newborn, since exposure to immunosuppression did occur. Early treatment of newborn infection is essential along with possible isolation from the mother due to the risk to her. Investigation of the possibility of adrenocortical insufficiency should be explored. Very little has been documented in the area of follow-up of the newborn of a transplant recipient. Evaluation of the offspring's status in later years with regard to fertility and immunity should be planned.

SUMMARY

It is important that the health care provider, especially the transplant coordinator, recognize the importance of his/her role as a resource person, an educator, and an advocate when caring for the young recipient

TABLE 7.5 Monitoring of Infants

- Electrolytes, kidney, and liver functions
- Congenital abnormalities
- Birth defects
- Susceptibility to infection
- General growth and maturity

who has become pregnant. Open channels of communication must be maintained. Addressing openly such issues as the patient's sexuality relieves the patient's hesitation to discuss such topics. Knowing when and how to discuss such subjects as amenorrhea, menstruation, loss of libido, and other fears the patient may have becomes an art on the part of the coordinator. The caregiver should not wait for the patient to bring such topics to the forefront, but should rather anticipate the patient's questions and initiate such discussions. The patient should be allowed to express her fears about her own limitations, including perhaps her distorted self-image due to surgical scars, or questions about ability to care for a young child. Ideally, the patient should be taught to be a part of her own care. She should be encouraged to ask questions and should be made to feel she is an active part of her own care as she tries to reestablish a near-normal lifestyle. The importance of effective planning when it comes to pregnancy must be emphasized. The healthier the mother, the greater is the chance of bringing a healthy infant into their new life.

ACKNOWLEDGMENT

Thanks to Drs. Raman Venkataramanan and Ashok Jain for their assistance in preparation of this chapter. Sincere thanks to my family for supporting my efforts.

REFERENCES

Bearn, A.G., Kunkel, H.G., & Slater, R.J. (1956). The problem of chronic liver disease in young women. *American Journal of Medicine, 21*, 3–15.

Becker, U. (1993). The influence of ethanol and liver disease on sex hormones and hepatic estrogen receptors in women. *Danish Medical Bulletin, 40,* 447–459.

Caplan, R. M., Dossetor, J. B., & Maughan, G. B. (1970). Pregnancy following cadaver kidney homotransplantation. *American Journal of Obstetrics and Gynecology, 106,* 644–648.

Cheng, Y.S. (1977). Pregnancy in liver cirrhosis and/or portal hypertension. *American Journal of Obstetrics and Gynecology, 128,* 812–822.

Cundy, T.F., O'Grady, J.G., & Williams, R. (1990). Recovery of menstruation and pregnancy after liver transplantation. *Gut, 31,* 337–338.

Davison, J. M. (1987). Renal transplantation and pregnancy. *American Journal of Kidney Diseases, 9,* 374–380.

Fair, J. A. S., Feng, T., Merritt, W. T., & Burdick, J. F. (1990). Intrapartum orthotopic liver transplantation with successful outcome of pregnancy. *Transplantation, 50,* 534–535.

Laifer, S. A., Darby, M. J., Scantlebury, V. P., Harger, J. H., & Caritis, S. N. (1990). Pregnancy and liver transplantation. *Obstetrics & Gynecology, 76,* 1083–1088.

Lau, R. J., & Scott, J. R. (1985). Pregnancy following renal transplantation. *Clinical Obstetrics and Gynecology, 28,* 339–350.

Lloyd, C. W., & Williams, R. H. (1948). Endocrine changes associated with Laënnec's cirrhosis of the liver. *American Journal of Medicine, 4,* 315–330.

Murray, J. E., Reid, D. E., Harrison, J. H., & Merrill, J. P. (1963). Successful pregnancies after human renal transplantation. *The New England Journal of Medicine, 269,* 341–343.

Penn, I., Makowski, E., Droegemueller, W., Halgrimson, C. G., & Starzl, T. (1971). Parenthood in renal homograft recipients. *Journal of the American Medical Association, 216,* 1755–1761.

Penn, I., Makowski, E. L., & Harris, P. (1980). Parenthood following renal and hepatic transplantation. *Transplantation, 30,* 397–400.

Scantlebury, V., Gordon, R., Tzakis, A., Koneru, B., Bowman, J., Mazzaferro, V., Stevenson, W. C., Todo, S., Iwatsuki, S., & Starzl, T. (1990). Childbearing after liver transplantation. *Transplantation, 49,* 317–321.

Sims, C. J., Porter, K. B., & Knuppel, R. A. (1989). Successful pregnancy after a liver transplant. *American Journal of Obstetrics and Gynecology, 161,* 532–533.

Walcott, W. O., Derick, D. E., Jolley, J. J., Schmid, R., & Snyder, D. L. (1978). Successful pregnancy in a liver transplant patient. *American Journal of Obstetrics and Gynecology, 132,* 340–341.

8

PREGNANCY AND BREAST-FEEDING WHILE RECEIVING CYCLOSPORINE A

Janet E. Madill, R.D., Gary Levy, M.D., and Paul Greig, M.D.

Female transplant recipients in the childbearing age group pose the questions: What are the effects of cyclosporine (CsA) on pregnancy? Will CsA be detrimental to the baby if the mother breast-feeds while taking this drug? CsA is a potent immunosuppressive agent that is highly metabolized, soluble, and extensively distributed in the body, causing many toxic side effects (Flechner, Katz, Rogers, Van Buren, & Kahan, 1985; Kossoy, Herbert, & Wentz, 1988; Venkataramanan et al., 1988). A major concern is whether these side effects will be potentiated in the fetus during gestation or in the baby after delivery, particularly when the mother is breast-feeding.

PART ONE: PREGNANCY AND CYCLOSPORINE

During the past decade, transplantation has become an acceptable treatment for end-stage disease of major organs. The majority of recipients rehabilitate to a normal lifestyle, and for the female patient, reproduction is a part of this normal process. The goal is for a safe, normal pregnancy and delivery.

Historical Perspective

Numerous studies have been published on pregnancy and immunosuppression. The following is a summary of the major results of these studies:

- Kossoy et al. (1988) discussed the management issues of heart transplant patients wishing to conceive. The authors focused on contraception, pregnancy, and risks to the mother and infant, among other issues. They concluded that pregnancy following heart transplantation while on CsA was acceptable with minimal side effects to the mother and infant.
- A case report was published by Lowenstein et al. (1988) on a heart transplant patient. The patient was diagnosed with chronic cardiomyopathy and received a heart transplant in November 1984. In 1986, the patient delivered a 1,450-gram infant at 31 weeks. She was controlled on 7.2 mg/kg/day of CsA and 16 mg prednisone/day. The authors concluded that this was a successful pregnancy with positive maternal and neonatal outcomes. Ahner, Kiss, and Zuckerman (1993) reported similar results.
- Tyden et al. (1989) reported four successful pregnancies in recipients of combined pancreas-kidney transplants. They concluded that successful conception and pregnancy could be obtained with good metabolic control throughout.
- A comprehensive overview was reported by Cockburn, Krupp, and Monka (1989) on 51 pregnancies in 48 renal transplant patients who received CsA during pregnancy. Their conclusions were that CsA did not induce any identifiable physical anomalies. They further reported that, although the drug crosses the placental barrier, there is no evidence of a direct hazard to the fetus.
- Madill, Tolton, Levy, and Greig (1990) published a complete review on pregnancy and immunosuppressive medications within the liver transplant population. That study reported on case studies up to 1989, which supported the conclusion that pregnancy was safe and acceptable following orthotopic liver transplantation while on CsA. Current literature continues to provide similar results (Baruch, Weiner, Enat, Ronen, & Blumenfield, 1993; Gunter, Mauz, Ringe, & Niesert, 1990; Haagsma, Klopmaker, Verwer, & Slooff, 1991; Madill, Taddio, Koren, Levy, & Greig, 1994).
- Aikin (1992) confirms that there are low risks to breast-feeding after

transplant and recommends a multidisciplinary approach to the management of pregnant heart-transplant patients.

- A study by Muirhead, Sabharwal, Rieder, Lazarovits, and Hollomby (1992) reported on 22 pregnancies in renal recipients. Risks to the offsprings were a high rate of prematurity, low birth weight, and intrauterine growth retardation (IUGR). Maternal risks included hypertension.
- Wagoner et al. (1993) reported on 29 infants born to heart and heart-lung recipients with minimal risks to the patient and offspring.
- Salmela, Kyllonen, Holmberg, and Gronhagen-Riska (1993) reported on 29 pregnancies in 22 renal recipients and 39 male recipients who fathered 65 children. They concluded a 70% 10-year survival rate in female recipients and reported no IUGR.
- Carmona et al. (1993) reported a successful pregnancy after a combined pancreas-kidney transplant.

Prenatal Issues

There is generalized agreement that women should avoid pregnancy for 12 to 24 months post-transplantation and should be in good metabolic control preconception (Armenti et al., 1994). The rationale for this is twofold. The incidence of acute rejection is highest within the first year following transplantation, and pregnancy may precipitate rejection. Moreover, after this period, the patient should be on the lowest dosage of immunosuppressive medications (Kirk, 1991). Armenti reported that maternal drug-treated hypertension, diabetes mellitus, and elevated serum creatinine may be predictors for loss of graft in pregnant kidney recipients.

Contraceptive Issues

Each method of birth control has its inherent problems and/or complications. Oral contraceptive agents (OCA) may cause thromboembolism and exacerbate CsA-induced hypertension (Kossoy et al., 1988). Moreover, OCAs may exacerbate coronary artery disease, seen in 40% of heart transplant recipients within 2 to 5 years following transplant. For these patients, OCAs may be contraindicated (Kossoy et al., 1988). However, new low-dose OCAs may not increase the risk of thromboembolism, and these should be considered (Kossoy et al., 1988). Intrauterine devices (IUDs) can increase the risk of infection and are therefore not recommended (Aikin, 1992; Kossoy et al., 1988). It appears that the barrier methods of contraception (including condoms, diaphragms, sponges, and foam) may be the safest alternatives (Aikin, 1992).

Pregnancy Issues

Although some authors suggest CsA does cross the placental barrier, it appears to pose no direct hazard to the fetus (Cockburn, Krupp, & Monka, 1989; Flechner et al., 1985; Kossoy et al., 1988). CsA has never been associated with consistent embryolethal or teratogenic effects (Cockburn et al., 1989; Kossoy et al., 1988; Ostensen, 1992) and did not produce any chromosomal abnormalities in animal studies (Venkataramanan et al., 1988).

Some researchers conclude a low placenta transfer of CsA due to its high molecular weight (Nandakumaran & Eldeen, 1990). However, there may be other complications seen in mothers and babies. These risks include preeclampsia (Wagoner et al., 1993), gestational diabetes (Tyden et al., 1989), hypertension (Scantlebury et al., 1990), prematurity and increased infections (Kossoy et al., 1988; Wagoner et al., 1993), intrauterine growth retardation (Flechner et al., 1985; Olshan, Mattison, & Zwanenburg, 1994; Ostensen, 1992), induction of a dormant cytomegalovirus (Kossoy et al., 1988), proteinuria, and an increased incidence of cesarean sections (Lowenstein et al., 1988). Other risks may be organ-specific; for example, pancreatic grafts placed too close to the uterus may compress the graft and induce pancreatitis as the pregnancy progresses (Tyden et al., 1989). There is some literature to indicate that twin pregnancies have occurred to women receiving CsA. The outcomes have been successful (Grow, Simon, Liss, & Delp, 1991; Wagoner et al., 1993).

Some literature suggests that children exposed to CsA in utero are at no risk for immunodeficiency or autoimmunity (Pilarski, Yacyshyn, & Lazarovits, 1994).

The distribution of lymphocytes returns to low-normal ranges within the first 2 years of life except for CD8 values, which may remain low (Baarsma & Kamps, 1993; Wagoner et al., 1993). However, these researchers concluded that there were no signs of persistent adverse effects of CsA on the immune system. Pregnancy can be considered an immunologically privileged state, evidenced by immunosuppressive medications being significantly reduced during this time without precipitating acute rejection (Wagoner et al., 1993). However, when the pregnancy is completed and the "immunologically privileged" state is over, baseline immunosuppressive medications should be reinstituted.

Labor and Delivery Issues

Immunosuppressed women should always be regarded as high-risk, and aseptic techniques during examination and delivery should be used (Aikin, 1992; Kossoy et al., 1988). Impaired wound healing with the use of immunosuppressive medications is well known. Cesarean sections would significantly increase the risks of infection and should be implemented only when absolutely necessary (Lowenstein et al., 1988).

Parental Issues

Despite the fact that CsA has changed the world of transplantation, there is still an uncertain life expectancy for these patients. The literature suggests that there is a 50% chance that male or female recipients will be alive when the child reaches 15 years (Kirk, 1991). Furthermore, there is some suggestion that female offspring may suffer some effect on their reproductive potential secondary to chronic immunosuppression in utero. This is currently speculation because there are no data to support this hypothesis (Scantlebury et al., 1990).

Conclusion

It has been recommended that women on CsA wait 1 to 2 years after their transplants to become pregnant. During this time, deciding which birth control method is most suitable and acceptable may present a challenge for the women and their health care providers. The risks and benefits of each method of birth control should be considered. Furthermore, the literature does suggest that it is safe for women on CsA to become pregnant, and the risks to the infant and mother should be fully discussed before conception.

PART TWO: BREAST-FEEDING AND CYCLOSPORINE

Mothers need to have the opportunity to breast-feed if they so choose. Recipients on CsA need to know whether breast-feeding is harmful to the baby.

Historical Perspective

Currently, very little research has been conducted on the safety of breast-feeding while taking CsA. The following are four reports on transplantation and breast-feeding:

- Coulam et al. (1982) reported two patients whose colostrum and/or breast milk were studied. Although the purpose of this study was to determine the level of another immunosuppressive agent in breast milk (azathioprine, not CsA), this study did conclude that, when the IgA levels in breast milk were examined, they were found to be similar in immunosuppressed and nonimmunosuppressed patients. Although this fact may seem insignificant, a full review and understanding of the immunological factors in breast milk changes its significance. It is known that breast milk does contain a wide range of protective factors including immunoglobulins, of which secretory IgA (sIgA) is the most significant (Whitehead, 1983). This is the only study that shows that immunosuppressed transplant women may still afford the ability to provide their infants with the much needed immunological factors.

- Lewis and Lamont (1983) reported a successful pregnancy of a 27-year-old female who was maintained on 450 mg/day of CsA. Although the mother did not breast-feed, CsA was detected in breast milk samples on days two (101 μg/L), three (109 μg/L), and four (263 μg/L) postpartum. An unpublished Sandoz document from 1982 showed that in animal studies CsA is excreted in breast milk in a maximum amount of 2% of the maternal dose. Based on this study and their findings of CsA in breast milk, the authors concluded that breast-feeding was contraindicated. The results of this study are difficult to interpret because maternal blood samples, milk samples, and the infant's blood CsA levels were not drawn simultaneously. Furthermore, the mother was not breast-feeding, and the levels of CsA may have been abnormally high because the breast was not continuously emptied.
- Grekas, Vasiliou, and Lazarides (1984) reported two pregnant renal transplant recipients who chose to breast-feed their infants despite being discouraged by the medical profession. They disclosed that, although immunosuppression drug levels in breast milk were not checked, the infants had normal blood cell counts, no increase in infections, and above-average growth rates.
- Flechner et al. (1985) reported on a 36-year-old renal allograft recipient. The patient was maintained on a daily dosage of 325 mg CsA and 10 mg of prednisone. A sample of breast milk obtained 22 hours after an oral dose of CsA contained 16 ng/ml of CsA. The CsA was assayed using a third-party mixed lymphocyte culture (MLC) suppression method. The authors did not discuss the correlation between levels of CsA in the mother, breast milk, and infant. Based on the fact that CsA was measurable in breast milk, their recommendation was to discourage breast-feeding.

The only literature available (Flechner et al., 1985; Lewis & Lamont, 1983) has suggested that it is not safe for mothers to breast-feed. They do not base the breast-feeding decision on data derived from a large clinical trial. Rather, they suggest that the mere presence of CsA in the breast milk may be deleterious to the infant and that, for this reason alone, mothers should be discouraged from breast-feeding (P. Y. Wong, personal communication, Feb. 1994).

The Toronto Hospital Experience

This study at the Toronto Hospital began with a worldwide literature review on CsA and its relationship to breast-feeding. The findings were compared to the clinical experiences of three recipients seen at our facility in 1989. For this study, CsA was measured using a high-performance liquid chromatographic method (Giesbrecht, Soldin, & Wong, 1989).

Case Report #1. In June 1988, a 33-year-old gravida II para II female underwent liver transplant for hepatic failure secondary to hepatitis C. She became pregnant 9 months later and was taking CsA, prednisone, and levothyroxine. The pregnancy was uneventful. On November 28, 1989, the patient underwent an elective cesarean section at 37 weeks and delivered a 3,030-gram male. Other than transient neonatal tachypnea, the infant did not experience any adverse events. The Apgar scores were 6 at 1 minute, 8 at 5 minutes, and 9 at 10 minutes. The infant had no signs of birth defects, metabolic toxicity, organ toxicity, or infection. The patient was taking 200 mg of CsA at 1000h and 2200h. Her trough blood CsA level taken at 0930h on the day before delivery (November 27) was 123 μg/L. A simultaneous colostrum level was 208 ug/L. Her last dose before delivery was at 2200h on November 27. On November 28, her colostrum CsA level taken at 1000h was 418 ug/L. (Her last dose of CsA was 2200h November 27.) Her 1100h blood level was 82 ug/L. The cord blood CsA level was 35 ug/L. The patient was discouraged from breast-feeding.

Case Report #2. A 17-year-old kidney transplant recipient in August 1988 became pregnant in 1989. At 34 weeks, she delivered a male on September 22, 1989. The baby was noted to have no anomalies. In July 1991, the patient received a second kidney transplant. She became pregnant again on January 31, 1993, and delivered via cesarean section a 32-week, 1,200-gram male. Her early delivery was performed due to impaired kidney function and proteinuria. The baby's Apgar scores were 6 at 1 minute and 8 at 5 minutes. There were no anomalies; however, the baby suffered from respiratory distress and was intubated immediately after birth. The neonate did well clinically and was extubated on February 4. Nasogastric feeding with formula commenced at this time. On February 5, the patient started methyldopa 500 mg TID for hypertension. The baby was given breast milk by nasogastric tube on February 6 and 7. The mother decided not to breast-feed. The baby was transferred to a periphery hospital and lost to further follow-up. Samples of maternal blood, colostrum, cord blood, and neonatal blood were tested for CsA content. At the time of delivery, the patient was taking CsA (150 mg twice daily at 1000h and 2200h) and prednisone (15 mg every other day). A maternal blood CsA level taken in the morning (1054h) on the day of delivery was 93 μg/L. A neonatal blood CsA level taken four days after delivery revealed a CsA level below the limit of detection of the assay (<15 μg/L); a maternal blood level taken the next day contained 134 μg/L of CsA. Five colostrum samples were obtained 3 to 5 days after delivery. The median CsA milk level was 99 μg/L (range, 36-209 μg/L).

Case Report #3. In August 1987, a 29-year-old, gravida 0 para 0 female underwent liver transplantation for hepatic failure secondary to hepatitis C. In April 1992, she became pregnant while taking prednisone, azathioprine, and CsA. The dosages of immunosuppressive therapy were modified throughout the course of the pregnancy. She delivered a 2,800-gram female at 38 weeks via cesarean section with no anomalies. The Apgar scores were 8 at 1 minute and 9 at 5 minutes. At the time of delivery, she was taking prednisone (10 mg daily), azathioprine (75 mg daily), and CsA (125 mg twice daily at 1000h and 2200h). Breast-feeding was adequately established until six days later, when breast-feeding was temporarily discontinued due to unnecessary concerns of potential toxicity to the neonate. Four days later the mother attempted to resume breast-feeding; however, inefficient neonatal suckling led to partial supplementation with formula.

Results

Maternal blood, milk, and neonatal blood samples were collected in the first few weeks postpartum and analyzed for CsA (see Table 8.1). On February 15, three weeks postpartum, the infant's BUN/creatinine were 44/2.5, both within the normal limits. Only one patient demonstrated the presence of 125 μg/L CsA in the mother, 45 μg/L in the breast milk, and 18 μg/L in the infant. (The 18 μg/L of CsA in the infant was considered a detectable but negligible amount because the limit of detection of an assay

TABLE 8.1 Longitudinal Study—Case Report #3: CsA Levels (μg/L).

	Maternal Blood		Maternal Milk		Infant Blood	
	Time	Level	Time	Level	Time	Level
*PP Day #1			22:50	58		
			—	56		
PP Day #3			—	57	12:00	18
PP Day #4	08:45	125	09:20	45		
	12:00	96	12:00	57		
	15:15	152	15:00	82		
	18:15	237	18:00	77		
PP Day #5					14:00	21
PP Day #6			05:27	137		
			11:45	105		
PP Day #9			22:40	130		
PP Day #10			05:35	203		
			12:28	164		
PP Day #21					13:50	21

Source: Toronto Hospital, 1993.
*PP = Postpartum.

was >15 μg/L.) Although the maternal milk CsA levels (Case Report #3) reached 200 μg/L, on postpartum day 10, the infant's blood CsA still remained in the detectable but negligible amount. This could reflect absorption and/or rapid metabolism, but at present this remains speculative. Long-term monitoring of the infant through blood tests indicated a normal BUN and creatinine, suggesting no renal toxicity. Thus, despite therapeutic levels of CsA in the mother's blood and mere comparable levels in maternal milk, it appears that the amount of CsA in the infant did not reach significant levels. In fact, the amount of CsA detected in the infant's blood was just minimally above background levels.

The infant showed no signs of renal or neural toxicity or hirsutism, which are the three most common side effects of CsA. Although one must caution the interpretation of a single case report, these results suggest that breast-feeding may be safe for mothers who have had transplants and are on CsA.

Conclusion

The Toronto Hospital transplant program's practice had been to advise mothers on immunosuppressive medications, in particular CsA, not to breast-feed. The rationale for this practice is now being reevaluated. However, an infant born to a woman on CsA who chooses to breast-feed must be closely monitored. Intensive monitoring involves measuring the mother's serum CsA and breast milk CsA and the infant's CsA levels as well as monitoring the infant for any possible toxic side effects. The amount of CsA that the infant is exposed to will depend on pharmacokinetic factors such as absorption distribution, metabolism, and elimination of CsA in the mother and baby.

Further research could focus on the long-term effects of CsA on the offspring of recipients. With close, careful follow-up and management, healthy outcomes for female transplant recipients and their offspring may be possible. An ethical issue, such as the uncertain life expectancy of the transplant recipients and the possibility that they may not live long enough to rear their children to adulthood, as well as the medical issues surrounding maternal and fetal welfare, must be considered on an individual basis. Much more research needs to be conducted relating to pregnancy and breast-feeding in transplant recipients.

EDITOR'S NOTE

In 1991, the National Transplantation Pregnancy Registry was established at Thomas Jefferson University in Philadelphia by a team whose principal investigator was Vincent T. Armenti, M.D., Ph.D. Initially, a questionnaire was distributed to 228 U.S. transplant centers. Another questionnaire was sent to female allograft recipients who had later become pregnant. This questionnaire asked about the lengths of their pregnancies, newborn birth weights and complications, immunosuppression, and presence of hypertension. A third questionnaire was sent to male recipients who had later fathered pregnancies. Many studies are being conducted on the data collected from these questionnaires. For further information, please contact the National Transplantation Pregnancy Registry at the following address:

Thomas Jefferson University Hospital
605 College Building
1025 Walnut Street
Philadelphia, PA 19107
Phone: (215) 955-2840

ACKNOWLEDGMENT

I wish to gratefully acknowledge all the effort and time that Antoinette Mattucci, research assistant at Toronto Hospital, has given to the development of this chapter.

REFERENCES

Ahner, R., Kiss, H., & Zuckerman, A. (1993). Pregnancy and spontaneous delivery 13 months after heart transplantation. *Geburtshilfe & Frauenheilkunde, 53,* 574–576.

Aikin, S. J. (1992). Pregnancy after heart transplantation. *Progress in Cardiovascular Nursing, 7,* 2–5.

Armenti, V. T., Ahlswede, K. M., Ahlswede, B. A., Jarrell, B. E., Moritz, M. J., & Burke, J. F. (1994). National Transplant Pregnancy Registry: Outcomes of 154 pregnancies in cyclosporine A-treated female kidney transplant recipients. *Transplantation, 57,* 502–506.

Baarsma, R., & Kamps, W. A. (1993). Immunological responses in an infant after cyclosporine A exposure during pregnancy. *European Journal of Pediatrics, 152,* 476–477.

Baruch, Y., Weiner, Z., Enat, R., Ronen, N., & Blumenfield, Z. (1993). Pregnancy after liver transplantation. *International Journal of Gynecology and Obstetrics, 41,* 273–276.

Carmona, F., Cararach, V., Bedini, J. L., Mas, E., Deulofeu, P., Ricart, M. J., & Fernandez-Cruz, L. (1993). Successful pregnancy after combined pancreas-kidney transplantation. *European Journal of Obstetrics, Gynecology, & Reproductive Biology, 52,* 143–145.

Cockburn, I., Krupp, P., & Monka, C. (1989). Present experience of Sandimmune in pregnancy. *Transplantation Proceedings, 21,* 3730–3732.

Flechner, S. M., Katz, A. R., Rogers, A. J., Van Buren, C., & Kahan, B. D. (1985). The presence of cyclosporine in body tissues and fluids during pregnancy. *American Journal of Kidney Disease, 5,* 60–63.

Giesbrecht, E. E., Soldin, S. J., & Wong, P. Y. (1989). A rapid, reliable high-performance liquid chromatographic micromethod for the measurement of cyclosporine in whole blood. *Therapeutic Drug Monitoring, 11,* 332–336.

Grekas, D. M., Vasiliou, S. S., & Lazarides, A. N. (1984). Immunosuppressive therapy and breast-feeding after renal transplantation. *Nephron, 37,* 128.

Grow, D. R., Simon, N. V., Liss, J., & Delp, W. T. (1991). Twin pregnancy after orthotopic liver transplantation, with exacerbation of chronic graft rejection. *American Journal of Perinatology, 8,* 135–138.

Gunter, H. H., Mauz, R., Ringe, B., & Niesert, S. (1990). Pregnancy following liver transplant and during immunosuppression with cyclosporine A. *Deutsche Medizinische Wochenschrift, 115,* 470–472.

Haagsma, E. B., Klopmaker, I. J., Verwer, R., & Slooff, M. J. (1991). Long-term results after liver transplantation in adults. *Scandinavian Journal of Gastroenterology, 188,* 38–43.

Kirk, E. P. (1991). Organ transplantation and pregnancy: A case report and review. *American Journal of Obstetrics and Gynecology, 164,* 1629–1633.

Kossoy, L. R., Herbert, C. M., & Wentz, A. C. (1988) Management of heart transplant recipients: Guidelines for the obstetrician-gynecologist. *American Journal of Obstetrics and Gynecology, 159,* 490–499.

Lewis, G. J., & Lamont, C. A. R. (1983). Successful pregnancy in a renal transplant recipient taking cyclosporin A. *British Medical Journal, 286,* 603.

Lowenstein, B. R., Vain, N. W., Perrone, S. V., Wright, D. R., Boullon, F. J., & Favaloro, R. G. (1988). Successful pregnancy and vaginal delivery after heart transplantation. *American Journal of Obstetrics and Gynecology, 158,* 589–590.

Madill, J., Taddio, A., Koren, G., Levy, G., & Greig, P. D. (1994, February). *Breastfeeding while receiving cyclosporin A.* (Paper presented at the meeting of the International Transplant Nurses Society, San Francisco, CA.)

Madill, J., Tolton, K., Levy, G., & Greig, P. D. (1990). The first baby born to a liver transplant recipient. *Transplantation/Implantation Today, 2,* 132.

Muirhead, N., Sabharwal, A. R., Rieder, M. J. Lazarovits, A. I., & Hollomby, D. J. (1992). The outcome of pregnancy following renal transplantation: The experience of a single centre. *Transplantation, 54,* 429–432.

Nandakumaran, M., & Eldeen, A. S. (1990). Transfer of cyclosporine A in the perfused human placenta. *Developmental Pharmacology and Therapeutics, 15,* 101–105.

Olshan, A. F., Mattison, D. R., & Zwanenburg, T. S. (1994). International commission for protection against environmental mutagens and carcinogens: Cyclosporine A: Review of genotoxicity and potential for adverse human reproductive and developmental effects: Reports of a working group on the genotoxicity of vyclosporine A. *Mutation Research, 317,* 163–173.

Ostensen, M. (1992). Treatment with immunosuppressive and disease modifying drugs during pregnancy and lactation. *American Journal of Reproductive Immunology, 28,* 148–152.

Pilarski, L. M., Yacyshyn, B. R., & Lazarovits, A. J. (1994). Analysis of peripheral blood lymphocyte populations and immune function from children exposed to cyclosporine A or azathioprine in utero. *Transplantation, 57,* 133–134.

Salmela, K. T., Kyllonen, L. E., Holmberg, C., & Gronhagen-Riska, C. (1993). Impaired renal function after pregnancy in renal transplant recipients. *Transplantation, 56,* 1372–1375.

Scantlebury, V., Gordon, R., Tzakis, A., Koneru, B., Bowman, J., Mazzaferro, V., Stevenson, W. C., Todo, S., Iwatsuki, S., & Starzl, T. E. (1990). Childbearing after liver transplantation. *Transplantation, 49,* 317–321.

Tyden, G., Brattstrom, C., Bjorkman, U., Landgraaf, R., Baltzer, J., Hillebrand, G., Land, W., Calne, R., Brons, I. G. M., Squifflet, J. P., Ghysen, J., & Alexandre,

G. P. J. (1989). Pregnancy after combined pancreas-kidney transplantation. *Diabetes, 38,* 43–45.

Venkataramanan, R., Koneru, B., Wang, C. P., Burckart, G. J., Caritis, S. N., & Starzl, T. E. (1988). Cyclosporine and its metabolites in mother and baby. *Transplantation, 46,* 468–469.

Wagoner, L., Taylor, D., Olsen, S. L., Price, G., Rasmussen, L. G., Larsen, C. B., Scott, J. R., & Renlund, D. G. (1993). Immunosuppressive therapy, management, and outcome of heart transplant recipients during pregnancy. *Journal of Heart and Lung Transplantation, 12,* 993–999.

Whitehead, R. G. (1983, Jan. 22). Nutritional aspects of human lactation. *Lancet,* 167–169.

PART IV
Economics of Transplantation

9

FEDERAL REGULATION OF TRANSPLANTATION: A TEN-YEAR PERSPECTIVE

Gwendolyn Mayes, B.A., M.S.

With passage of the National Organ Transplant Act of 1984 (NOTA) the federal government began the process of establishing a comprehensive framework for the development and implementation of transplantation policy that would bring together organ procurement organizations and transplant centers within one national coordinated system (Notice of Proposed Rulemaking, 1994). Transplantation professionals sought expanded funding coverage for new immunosuppressive therapies with heart and liver transplantation. Once awakened to these issues, Congress became interested in the lack of a national system to register transplant patients (Dennis, 1992). Other concerns, such as equal access to trans-

DISCLAIMER: This chapter was written by Ms. Mayes in her individual capacity. The views expressed in this chapter do not necessarily reflect the views of the Department of Health and Human Services or the Federal Government.

plantation, the lack of donor organs, and the possibility of profiteering in organ exchange were of interest to Congress and helped build momentum for passing federal legislation. Key provisions of the NOTA were as follows:

- It required the establishment of a national task force to conduct a comprehensive review of the medical, legal, ethical, social, and economic issues.
- It authorized funds for grants to organ procurement organizations (OPOs) for the primary purpose of consolidating existing entities or establishing new organizations.
- It required the establishment of the National Organ Procurement and Transplantation Network (OPTN).
- It required the establishment of a scientific registry of transplant patients.
- It created an entity within the Public Health Service (of the U.S. Department of Health and Human Services, hereafter "Department") to administer the law and to carry out a program of public education regarding the need for increased donations.

One additional major provision of the act was its ban of the purchase or sale of human organs. While its regulatory history is relatively sparse, this provision was Congress' reaction to the prevailing concern that a "market" approach to transplantation would emerge. This ban, one of the first federal regulatory measures concerning transplantation that was unrelated to the federal government's role as payer, continues to shape transplant policy by limiting the options available for testing incentives (e.g., financial and others) which would possibly increase donation (Blumstein, 1989). Others have noted that it is inconsistent for a society to prohibit the sale of organs and then distribute them according to the ability to pay, arguing that it is difficult to distinguish buying an organ for transplantation from buying an organ transplant procedure when the organ is provided with the procedure (Beauchamp & Childress, 1989). The prohibition did not, however, include the reasonable payment associated with removal, transportation, implantation, processing, etc., of a human organ in connection with the donation (*Conference Report 98-1127*, 1984).

Section 301 of the National Organ Transplant Act added a provision that prohibited the purchase or sale of any organ for use in transplantation. The provision reads, "(a) it shall be unlawful for any person to knowingly acquire, receive, or otherwise transfer any human organ for valuable consideration for use in human transplantation if the transfer affects interstate commerce. Any person who violates subsection (a) shall be fined not more than $50,000 or imprisoned not more than five years, or both."

TASK FORCE ON ORGAN TRANSPLANTATION

The original Transplant Act mandated the establishment of a Task Force to conduct comprehensive examinations of the medical, legal, ethical, economic, and social issues presented by human organ procurement and transplantation and to report recommendations for these issues (Task Force on Organ Transplantation, 1986). The composition of the Task Force included physicians and scientists; federal officials; and individuals with expertise in law, theology, ethics, health care financing, and social behavior.

RECOMMENDATIONS

During a period of 15 months, the national task force considered a wide range of topics. Their report, issued in 1986, contained over 70 recommendations targeted to legislative bodies, government agencies, professional organizations, and the general public. The task force adopted the position that organs are donated in a spirit of altruism and volunteerism and constitute a national resource to be used for the public good (Task Force on Organ Transplantation, 1986). Various approaches to increasing organ donation were proposed; important among these was the recommendation that required request/routine referral legislation be enacted in all states (Task Force on Organ Transplantation, 1986).

The task force also recommended that a set of explicit criteria be used by the Health Care Financing Administration to designate transplant centers. At the time of the report, there was a growing concern regarding the flurry of new transplant centers (see Table 9.1) and the implications of this development for organ allocation and patient care. It was believed that the proliferation of transplant centers would diminish the overall level of expertise, since there seemed to be a limited number of cadaver donors available (Jonasson, 1987). In recent years, survival data have been sufficient to analyze the volume effect on transplant outcomes. Recent studies in cardiac transplantation, for example, indicate that the risk of mortality at early and intermediate time points (1 and 12 months) increases by 40.3% and 33.1%, respectively, in centers performing fewer than nine cardiac transplants per year (Hosenpud, Breen, Edwards, Daily, & Hunsicker, 1994). The Task Force also urged the private sector to establish criteria for the reimbursement of transplant procedures that were based on experience, logistic medical support, volume, and graft and patient survival (Task Force on Organ Transplantation, 1986).

TABLE 9.1 Number of Transplant Centers by Organ

	1984	1987	1990	1993
Heart	37	123	148	164
Kidney	170	199	232	246
Liver	25	59	85	112
Pancreas	8	24	63	112
Heart-Lung	4	18	79	89
Lung	0	18	68	76
Total	244	441	675	799

Sources: Adapted from data from Battelle-Seattle Research Center, Seattle, Washington; United Network for Organ Sharing, Richmond, Virginia; Health Care Financing Administration, Baltimore, Maryland.

Over the past decade, recommendations of the Task Force on Organ Transplantation have been used as the "blueprint" for transplant activities. Questions relating to increasing donation, reimbursement, organ sharing, coordinating research, and immunosuppressive treatments have all, at one time or another, referenced the task force report. Many of the recommendations have been accomplished; others need to be implemented.

THE ORGAN PROCUREMENT AND TRANSPLANTATION NETWORK

The cornerstone of the NOTA and a central issue for the task force was the establishment of the Organ Procurement and Transplantation Network (OPTN). The House report (H. Rep. No. 98–575, 1983) that accompanied the legislation stated that the House Committee intended for the OPTN to be a strong, active national network for matching donated organs. Further, Congress stated that the responsibilities for coordinating the activities of the OPTN should be located in the private sector rather than in the federal government, one of the ways in which the act most deviated from a purely regulatory approach (Blumstein, 1989). In fiscal year 1986, $379,200 was awarded to the United Network for Organ Sharing (UNOS) for a one-year contract. UNOS, a private nonprofit organization, already maintained a voluntary transplant recipient registry and computer matching system (Sundwall, 1987). Another $1.2 million was awarded in September 1987 for, among other purposes, merging the computer capabilities and data collection of UNOS with another existing computer registry for nonrenal transplants maintained by the North

American Transplant Coordinators Organization. The OPTN contract was competitively awarded to UNOS in September 1990 for 3 years and again in September of 1993 (United Network for Organ Sharing [UNOS], 1994a).

Essentially, the goal of the OPTN was, and continues to be, the establishment and maintenance of a single, computerized, national waiting list for the matching of organs with potential recipients. At the time the OPTN became fully operational in the fall of 1987, there were approximately 13,000 patients waiting for transplants, a number that has nearly tripled in recent years (see Table 9.2). The OPTN was considered to be the authoritative body for transplant policymaking in the U.S. and responsible for determining national goals, setting policies, and monitoring the performance of its members (Mayes, 1992). At the helm was its board of directors representing various transplant professions, patients, and the general public. The board was charged with developing policies and procedures for membership in the OPTN, the allocation of donor organs, and ways to minimize organ wastage. Then Senator Albert Gore, Jr., a leading voice in transplant legislation, remarked the following:

> By giving those on the front lines (transplant professionals, patients) the authority to set policy, and by backing them up with the enforcement tools traditionally reserved for the bureaucracy, we sought a new way to streamline the process of setting policy. (Gore, 1989)

With the enactment of the Omnibus Budget Reconciliation Act of 1986 (OBRA '86), however, membership in the OPTN was no longer voluntary

TABLE 9.2 Number of Patients Waiting for Transplantation at End of Each Year, 12/31/84–12/31/94

	1984	*1987	1988	1989	1990	1991	1992	1993
Heart	100	646	1,030	1,320	1,788	2,267	2,690	2,834
Kidney	8,562	11,872	13,943	16,294	17,883	19,352	22,376	24,973
Liver	300	450	616	827	1,237	1,676	2,323	2,997
Pancreas	30	37	163	320	473	600	126	183
Kidney-Pancreas	N/A	N/A	N/A	N/A	N/A	N/A	778	923
Heart-Lung	N/A	148	205	240	225	154	180	202
Lung	N/A	14	69	94	308	670	942	1,240
Total	8,430	13,167	16,026	19,095	21,914	24,719	29,415	33,352

*Data for 1985 and 1986 were incomplete and therefore not included in this table.
Sources: Adapted from Battelle-Seattle Research Center, Seattle, Washington; United Network for Organ Sharing, Richmond, Virginia; Health Care Financing Administration, Baltimore, Maryland.

but a mandatory condition for Medicare– and Medicaid–participating hospitals that performed organ transplants. A new Section 1138 of the Social Securities Act required transplant centers to be members of and abide by the rules and requirements of the OPTN in order to qualify for Medicare or Medicare payments (Notice of Proposed Rulemaking, 1988). These rules included such things as physician training, laboratory standards, and organ allocation. Section 1138 was intended to protect transplant patients by assuring equitable access to the limited supply of organs and by assuring that transplants are performed in accordance with acceptable medical practice (H. Rep. No. 100–383, 1987).

Following the enactment of OBRA '86, discussions arose regarding the authority of a private contractor to issue substantive rules, enforced by the federal government, without any direct federal control or accountability, and in the absence of meaningful public participation (Lawton, 1989). At the center of the discussion was the unresolved issue of the extent of the OPTN's authority for establishing transplant policy. Thus, what originated as a purely voluntary process became a mandatory requirement for Medicare and Medicaid hospitals' access to public funding. For some it made for an unusual, if not somewhat troublesome, public-private relationship. While it is extraordinary for a private contractor to assert authority on behalf of the government (Lawton, 1989), challenges to its constitutionality have been unsuccessful.

In response to the concerns raised regarding Section 1138, the Department of Health and Human Services published a general notice in the *Federal Register* in 1989 announcing its policy regarding this matter. It stated the following:

> In order to be a rule or requirement of the OPTN, and therefore mandatory or binding on hospitals and OPOs participating in Medicare or Medicaid, the Secretary (of the Department) must have given formal approval to the rule or requirement. No hospital will be considered out of compliance with the regulations (for participation) unless the Secretary has given the OTPN formal notice approving the decision to exclude the entity from the OPTN and has also notified the entity in writing. (Notice of Proposed Rulemaking, 1994)

With this action, the department took the position that OPTN policies were akin to Medicare conditions of participation and thus were subject to the same rulemaking procedures as required by the Administrative Procedures Act. The department reinforced its concern that OPTN policies, which were binding on its members, did not conflict with or exceed federal standards.

In late 1988, the Organ Transplant Amendments (amending the NOTA) were signed by President Reagan. They included provisions that the

OPTN "establish membership criteria and medical criteria for allocating organs and provide to members of the public an opportunity to comment with respect to such criteria" (H. Rep. No. 100–383, 1987). Congress clearly intended that the OPTN policies reflect a broad consensus of expert medical judgment and that these policies be developed openly, with full opportunity for participation by all interested parties and the public. The OPTN was encouraged to arrange for public comment at least once a year, even if no policy changes were proposed. Even though OPTN policies were to be developed by a private contractor, it was intended that they mirror the federal government's process of promulgating regulations as closely as possible (H. Rep. No. 100–383). Congress' interest in increasing public participation in the OPTN policymaking process was again a central issue in the reauthorization of the transplant act in 1990. The OPTN board composition was restructured in hopes of providing greater continuity in leadership and increased public accountability (Sen. Rep. No. 101–530, 1990).

During the 1990 reauthorization, Congress noted its "deep concern" for the manner in which the OPTN had functioned, citing additional concerns regarding the significant amount of time that had passed since the issuance of the department's 1989 policy decision that required formal departmental review and approval of OPTN policies. Simply stated, Congress felt that a policy vacuum had been created and urged the Department to proceed with publishing regulations (Sen. Rep. No. 101–530).

As noted above, in keeping with the department's policy and Congress' intent that policies undergo a full public comment process, the department issued a "Notice of Proposed Rulemaking" (NPRM) on September 8, 1994, for the purpose of proposing a framework for the operation of the OPTN. The proposed rules provide for federal oversight of the *processes* by which the OPTN establishes policies, especially as they relate to the allocation of organs for transplant (Notice of Proposed Rulemaking, 1994). Public participation in OPTN policy development was emphasized. The NPRM also created an enforceable standard that OPTN member transplant programs must meet to qualify to receive organs for transplantation. Issuance of the proposed rule reinforced the federal government's ultimate and final control over the activities of the OPTN. For example, the Secretary would be able to object to any OPTN policy and direct the OPTN to revise the policy. In addition, hospitals denied transplant center designation and thus denied access to organs for transplantation would be able to appeal to the Secretary of Health and Human Services, and the OPTN must comply with the Secretary's final decision (Mayes, 1994).

GRANT PROGRAM FOR INCREASING DONATION

An important provision in the original transplant act was the authorization of a grant program for the purpose of increasing the availability of donor organs. The goals of the program were to provide organ procurement services in geographical areas without such services, to find ways of improving the efficiency and productivity of existing OPOs, and to consolidate organ procurement services in areas where there were multiple, and therefore potentially duplicative, OPOs (Sundwall, 1987). Then, as now, the limited number of donors (see Table 9.3) and the shortage of organs for transplantation hampered the rate of transplantation nationwide (Randall, 1991). This trend has continued in recent years, despite studies indicating the possibility of increasing the number of donors in the U.S. by 80% (Evans, Orains, & Ascher, 1992) and extensive efforts to educate the public (Novello, Braslow, & Mayes, 1992). Although the total number of donors (cadaveric and living) has grown over the past decade from 5,908 donors in 1988 to 7,099 donors in 1992, growth since 1990 has been due primarily to the increased use of living donors (Bennett, Glascock, Breen, Ellison, & Daily, 1993).

The first grants, originally limited to OPOs, were awarded in 1986. Eighteen grantees received a total of $1.9 million for a variety of planning and consolidation activities, primarily to avoid duplication of efforts. Through 1989 and 1994, a special goal of the grant program was to increase minority donation. This was a result of a relatively low donation rate among minority populations and studies that indicated that African-

TABLE 9.3 Number of Cadaveric Organ Donors, 1984–1993

Year	Number of Donors
1984	3,290
1985	3,637
1986	3,990
1987	4,000
1988	4,083
1989	4,016
1990	4,515
1991	4,530
1992	4,521
1993	4,845

Sources: Adapted from data from United Network for Organ Sharing, Richmond, Virginia; Health Care Financing Administration, Baltimore, Maryland.

TABLE 9.4 Grant Activity, 1986–1994

Fiscal Year	Number of Grants Awarded	Total Dollar Amount
1994	1	$100,000
1993	4	$337,648
1992	10	$401,000
1991	9	$308,000
1990	8	$492,000
1989	9	$485,000
1988	18	$1,300,000
1987	18	$2,700,000
1986	18	$2,000,000

Source: Adapted from data from Division of Organ Transplantation, Grants to Increase Organ Donation, 1986–1994.

Americans spend longer times on the kidney waiting list than Caucasians (Grant Compendium, 1992). In total, the department has awarded 95 grants totaling approximately $8.1 million (see Table 9.4). Even though the grant program has been included in each reauthorization of the transplant act, in recent years the size of the appropriation has been considerably less than in the earlier years of the program.

SCIENTIFIC REGISTRY OF TRANSPLANT RECIPIENTS

The transplant act required the department to establish a registry to collect data for the continuous evaluation of the clinical and scientific status of transplantation in the U.S. In 1984, organ-specific registries existed for heart, liver, kidney, bone marrow, and pancreas; however, they were strictly voluntary and did not include national data. UNOS was awarded the first Scientific Registry contract in September 1987 and chose to subcontract to existing registries for the collection of most data. UNOS was again awarded the contract through competitive processes in 1990 and 1993. In contrast to the OPTN, which collects data on pretransplant activities (e.g., donors and transplant candidates), the Scientific Registry collects post-transplant recipient data from the time of transplant until 2 years following graft failure or recipient death (United Network for Organ Sharing, 1994b). The data have been used in a variety of ways, the most important of which is to support transplant policy decisions. Examples of specific issues that have been addressed using the database include the following:

- The impact of antigen matching on transplant outcomes;
- the impact of various organ preservation methods on outcome;
- differential patient and graft survival rates among transplant programs; and
- transplant outcomes as a function of patient status and disease diagnosis (United Network for Organ Sharing, 1994a).

With an increasing number of transplant procedures performed each year (see Table 9.5), the number of patients followed through the Scientific Registry has grown considerably. Medical and scientific data on approximately 100,000 patients have been collected by UNOS since 1987, and data on thousands more (transplanted prior to the award of the national contract) have been added by organ-specific registries and the federal government (T. J. Breen, personal communication, Nov. 1994). This rich source of information provides the transplant community, private researchers, and the federal government with the most comprehensive data available for determining specific ways in which policies can be developed to maximize the number of transplants, graft survival, and equity in organ allocation (United Network for Organ Sharing, 1994b).

RECENT ACTIVITIES

The National Organ Transplant Act was scheduled for reauthorization in 1993; however, House and Senate bills died in conference, primarily due to unexpected hurdles created by Congress' increasing interest with health care reform. Although hearings were held, contentious issues such as whether or not OPOs and donor hospitals should have exclusive agreements and whether organs should be allocated within certain geographic areas added to the demise of the bill (Desmarais, 1993). The program received, however, an appropriation of $2,629,000 for fiscal year 1995. Regardless of specific legislation action, the implications for transplantation under an increasingly structured and premanaged system of health care are extensive. More and more transplant centers will have to operate under fixed budgets by capitation and case rates (Studin, 1993). Third-party payers, such as health maintenance organizations, may limit the number of transplant centers they contract to do business with, and those centers without managed care contracts will be vulnerable. Quality and efficiency will be critical success factors for designated transplant centers, and center-specific and procedure-specific data will be used liberally to evaluate performance (Studin, 1993). In this area, transplant professionals

TABLE 9.5 Number of Transplant Procedures Performed in the United States, 1984–1993

	1984	1985	1986	1987	1988	1989	1990	1991	1992	1993
Heart	346	719	1,368	1,512	1,676	1,705	2,108	2,126	2,169	2,299
Kidney*	6,968	7,695	8,976	8,967	9,043	8,988	9,877	10,102	10,232	10,931
Liver	308	602	924	1,182	1,713	2,201	2,691	2,953	3,064	3,442
Pancreas	87	112	170	180	249	417	528	531	557	771
Heart-Lung	N/A	30	42	41	33	93	203	405	535	665
Lung	N/A	20	N/A	11	74	67	52	51	48	60
Total	7,709	9,178	11,480	11,893	12,788	13,471	15,459	15,637	16,605	18,168

*Includes kidneys from cadaveric donors and living related kidney transplants.
Sources: Adapted from data from Battelle-Seattle Research Center, Seattle, Washington; United Network for Organ Sharing, Richmond, Virginia; Health Care Financing Administration, Baltimore, Maryland.

have taken a leading role by reporting center-specific patient and graft survival rates in 1991 and 1994 (United Network for Organ Sharing, 1991, 1994b). Ultimately, however, trends in managed care have the potential to limit the growth or even reduce the number of transplant centers (Sofaer, 1994).

CONCLUSION

When the National Organ Transplant Act passed in 1984, it received the endorsement of virtually every medical and scientific organization involved in organ transplantation. While Congress' attention was initially focused on funding for immunosuppressive drugs and certain extrarenal transplant procedures, further review and testimony bore forth the need to establish a national system so that transplants were available not only to those who primarily had the resources (access to publicity, fundraising) to receive priority. Coordinating existing efforts, especially in the area of organ procurement and transplant services, was of paramount importance.

The transplant act provided a national network to coordinate activities, a grant program to increase organ donation, a registry to collect data, and a task force charged with investigating and reporting on related issues. However, what began as a voluntary effort to *coordinate* activities soon became more regulatory in nature with the subsequent legislation in 1986 and 1988. Within the same year that the OPTN and Scientific Registry became fully operational, questions arose about the role of a private contractor (albeit charged by legislation and contract to do so) to establish policies and procedures that could determine a hospital's participation in federal funding programs. A federal notice has only recently been issued to receive public comment on this arrangement. In the interim, even though OPTN policies are considered voluntary, the level of participation, compliance, and accountability among OPTN members is extraordinary. This is particularly true in relation to organ allocation, a difficult and challenging area in which to reach consensus. With an increasing number of patients being listed for transplantation and few increases in the number of donors, decisions regarding who should receive a transplant have become more difficult over time.

Today, differing opinions on how to allocate organs equitably monopolize discussions on a national level, often overshadowing efforts to increase donation (Sen. Rep. No. 103–233, 1994). In contrast, "allocation" was mentioned only once in the conference report that accompanied the original transplant act (*Conference Report 98–1127*, 1984). Increasingly, transplant patients, their families, and the general public are being asked to participate in allocation decisions. The National Organ Transplant Act, now 10 years old, remains the cornerstone on which transplant policy is based. Future amendments will need to reflect the dynamic and often controversial challenges that surround this area of medicine.

ACKNOWLEDGMENT

The author wishes to gratefully acknowledge the assistance of Ms. Judith B. Braslow and Mr. Stephen Smolinski in the preparation of this manuscript.

REFERENCES

Beauchamp, T. L., & Childress, J. F. (1989). *Principles of biomedical ethics.* New York: Oxford University Press.

Bennett, L. E., Glascock, R. F., Breen, T. J., Ellison, M. D., & Daily, O. P. (1993). Organ donation in the United States: 1988 through 1992. In P. Terasaki (Ed.), *Clinical transplants* (pp. 85–93). Los Angeles: UCLA Tissue Typing Laboratory.

Blumstein, J. F. (1989, Feb.). *Government's role in transplantation policy.* Presentation to the National Health Lawyers Association, Legal Aspects of Organ Transplantation, Washington, DC.

Conference Report No. 98–1127, 98th Cong., 2nd Sess. (1984).

Dennis, J. M. (1992). A review of centralized rule-making in American transplantation. *Transplantation Reviews, 6,* 130-137.

Desmarais, H. R. (1993). A report from Washington. *The Chimera, 5,* 3.

Evans, R.W., Orains, C. E., & Ascher, N. L. (1992). The potential supply of organ donors: An assessment of the efficiency of organ procurement efforts in the United States. *Journal of the American Medical Association, 267,* 239-246.

Final rule: Medicare and Medicaid programs. (1988, March 1). *Federal Register, 53*(40), 6526–6551.

Gore, A. (1989, October 16). Remarks. Institute of Medicine Annual Meeting, Washington, DC.

Grant Compendium. (1992). Division of Organ Transplantation, U.S. Department of Health and Human Services.

Hearing on organ transplantation program: Hearings before the Subcommittee on Health and the Environment, 100th Cong., 1st Sess. (1987) (testimony of Olga Jonasson).

Hosenpud, J. D., Breen, T. J., Edwards, E. B., Daily, O. P., & Hunsicker, L. G. (1994). The effect of transplant center volume on cardiac transplant outcome. *Journal of the American Medical Association, 271,* 1844-1849.

H. Rep. No. 98–575. (1983). Committee on Energy and Commerce, 98th Cong., 1st Sess.

H. Rep. No. 100–383. (1987). Committee on Energy and Commerce, 100th Cong., 1st Sess.

Lawton, S. E. (1989, February). *UNOS and the public interest.* Presentation to The National Health Lawyers Association, Washington, DC.

Mayes, G. (1992, May). *The body and its parts as property: Ownership, donation and the sale of organs.* Presentation to Johns Hopkins School of Public Health Conference on Ethical Issues in Public Health, Baltimore, Maryland.

Mayes, G. (1994). *Summary: Notice of proposed rulemaking for organ procurement and transplantation regulations.* Supplement to J. Warren (Ed.), *Transplant News,* Washington, DC.

Notice of Proposed Rulemaking: Organ Procurement and Transplantation Network. (1994, September 8). *Federal Register, 59*(173), 46482–46499.

Novello, A. C., Braslow, J. B., & Mayes, G. (1992). Increasing organ donation: A report from the Surgeon General's workshop. *Journal of the American Medical Association, 267,* 213.

Randall, T. (1991). Too few human organs for transplantation, too many in need . . . and the gap widens. *Journal of the American Medical Association, 265,* 1223–1224.

Section 301 of the National Organ Transplant Act, Section 301 of Public Law 98-507 (42USC 274e)

Sen. Rep. No. 101–530. (1990). Committee on Labor and Human Resources, 101st Cong., 2nd Sess.

Sen. Rep. No. 103–233. (1994). Committee on Labor and Human Resources, 103rd Cong., 2nd Sess.

Sofaer, S. (1994, February). *Health care reform and managed competition: Restructuring health services.* Paper presented at the Division of Organ Transplantation Annual Meeting, Washington, DC.

Studin, I. (1993, October). *Managed care and its impact on transplantation.* Paper presentation at First National Transplant Policy Forum, Washington, DC.

Sundwall, D. N. (1987, March). *Federal efforts to improve the organ procurement system.* Paper presented at Pediatric Brain Death and Tissue Retrieval Conference sponsored by the American Council on Transplantation, Washington, DC.

Task Force on Organ Transplantation. (1986). *Transplantation: Issues and recommendations.* Washington, DC: U.S. Department of Health and Human Services.

United Network for Organ Sharing (UNOS). (1991). *Report of center-specific graft and patient survival rates.* Richmond, VA: Author.

United Network for Organ Sharing (UNOS). (1994a). *Annual Report.* Richmond, VA: Author.

United Network for Organ Sharing (UNOS). (1994b). Report of center-specific graft and patient survival rates. Richmond, VA: Author.

10

ECONOMIC TRENDS IN CALIFORNIA HEALTH CARE FOR TRANSPLANTATION

Laura L. Adams, B.S.

THE BEGINNINGS OF CONTRACTING

The term "center of excellence" is often used casually by hospital program development staff to describe a program in which the hospital has comparatively outstanding clinical strength and to which it has devoted additional service and marketing resources—a market leader. In the field of transplantation and other highly specialized procedures, the term has a much more specific meaning:

> A center of excellence is a facility that has performed a specialized procedure with enough frequency to become expert, thereby reducing morbidity and mortality. To encourage the patient volume needed to maintain their expert status, these centers are generally willing to give discounted prices to make it worthwhile for payors to send patients great distances to receive care. The theory is that patients will receive better care than at their local hospitals, and at lower costs. (Traska, 1989, p. 16)

The concept of competitively contracting for transplant services through nationally identified centers of excellence would significantly alter the future of solid organ and bone marrow transplant programs across the nation, turning what was once a research- and clinically driven technological advancement into a fiercely competitive tertiary and quaternary hospital service. However, when insurance giants such as Prudential, United Healthcare, and John Hancock first instituted centers of excellence transplant networks in the late 1980s, they attracted relatively little notice from hospitals and other health care providers (Koska, 1990).

While the overall price tag to the consumer and insurance companies for transplant services has historically been deemed extremely high, prior to the overall advent of managed care and centers of excellence in particular, little attention was given by providers to the overall cost, and resulting charges, of providing such care. In addition, prior to the late 1980s, the relative infrequency of transplants led payors to view these cases as exceptions—simply put, the catastrophic case. Payors reimbursed hospitals and physicians for transplant services (when deemed nonexperimental) at a minimal percent discount from total billed charges. Thus, from a hospital's economic standpoint, high charges and minimal discounts translated to a financially lucrative transplant program.

With payors now seeking new strategies to reduce costs, transplants became an ideal launching place for management both from a cost and an outcome perspective (Taylor, 1994). Although the overall incidence of transplantation was relatively small, representing a statistically small risk to the payor, charges for even one of these procedures often created significant financial liability. Additionally, as transplantation became less experimental and as new transplant types were evolving, payors recognized that their overall financial risk for transplantation would increase as the number of transplants increased (see Table 10.1). Payors sought to identify variance in outcomes between transplant programs, hoping to assure themselves and their employer clients that they were receiving the best possible outcomes for the most reasonable price.

Centers of excellence contracting radically altered the way in which hospitals with high-tech, high-dollar transplant programs would receive and be reimbursed for patients. The goal of the payors was to develop a set of minimum clinical criteria by which to review, select, and contract with a limited number of transplant programs. Payors redesigned their benefit plans to incorporate significant financial incentives to direct patients to contracted transplant programs. Payors requested (and received) significant discounts from the selected hospital and transplant surgeons/physicians because, in theory, they would be directing more volume to contracted programs.

TABLE 10.1 Increase in Number of Transplant Procedures Since 1988

	1988	1989	1990	1991	1992	1993
Liver	1,713	2,201	2,691	2,953	3,064	3,443
Kidney						
Cadaveric	7,232	7,086	7,782	7,734	7,695	8,168
Living-related donor	1,812	1,902	2,095	2,369	2,537	2,752
Pancreas	249	417	528	531	557	771
Heart	1,675	1,705	2,108	2,126	2,169	2,298
Heart-Lung	74	67	52	51	48	60
Lung	33	93	203	405	534	664
BMT*	3,263	4,034	4,484	5,150	5,770+	6,300+
Total	16,227	17,592	19,838	20,941	21,829	23,697

Sources: Adapted from United Network for Organ Sharing (UNOS), Published Statistics, 1994.
*Hauboldt, R. *Research Report—Cost Implications of Human Organ Transplantation, an Update: 1993.* Milliman & Robertson, Inc. 1993.
+Estimated

CONTRACTING

The first inkling that Stanford University Medical Center (now known as Stanford Health Services) had entered into a fierce national competition for payor accounts was in 1990, when a letter was received by Stanford from Travelers Insurance Company. The following excerpt exemplifies the change in contracting concepts:

> In expanding our commitment to provide quality and cost-effective employee health benefits, The Travelers is developing a national "Centers of Excellence" program for use by all Travelers subscribers and clients. This program will enhance Travelers customers' access to providers with recognized expertise in performing certain complex medical and surgical procedures. The initial phase of the program will involve our formation of select partnerships with leading major organ and tissue transplantation facilities. (G. Strong, communication to Specialty Contracting Department, 1990)

Establishing their own clinical criteria for participation in their network, payors sent out extensive clinical questionnaires to transplant programs across the nation. The questionnaire, or Request for Proposal (RFP), routinely included queries concerning volumes, survival rates, and morbidity for each adult and pediatric transplant program at the facility.

It also typically asked about program longevity, willingness of the program and hospital to participate in the payors' continuous quality improvement efforts, and evaluation of physician staff credentials.

For the first time, transplant programs found themselves in the unique and unsettling position of having to provide both outcome and programmatic data to an outside entity for review. In effect, the programs were required to *qualify* both in terms of meeting the established clinical criteria, and in agreeing to the "right" price. Moreover, most transplant programs were neither staffed nor prepared to complete the lengthy RFPs. These factors, often combined with institutional and programmatic beliefs that third-party payors would not be successful in such selective contracting and aggressive pricing, led many medical centers, at least initially, to ignore the RFPs in the belief that transplant programs would continue to thrive without such participation.

As Prudential, Hancock, and others began the tedious process of establishing their initial national networks, some large, prominent transplant programs found themselves in the unlikely position of being excluded from participation. Usually this exclusion resulted from one of two causes: Either the program had neglected to complete the RFP, or it failed to meet the clinical and outcome criteria that had been established for participation. Other factors influencing nonselection often included price competitiveness and political considerations.

However, no single event could have generated the kind of "wake-up call" that noninclusion turned out to be. When calling for an authorization to evaluate a patient, transplant center staff would find themselves advised that their transplant program was not participating in that particular transplant network, and the patient would be redirected to another facility. In the early 1990s, with managed care continuing to evolve and increasing numbers of payors instituting "centers of excellence," it became clear that participation in centers of excellence networks could spell the survival or failure of a transplant program.

The process for participating in a "centers of excellence" transplant network typically involves the following stages:

Phase 1: Facility Completes and Returns Request for Proposal (RFP), Containing Clinical and Administrative Questions Related to:

- Hospital licensure, malpractice coverage, utilization management program, quality assurance activities
- Program-specific data on volumes, survival, complications, retransplant rates, infection and rejection rates

- Staffing information on each unit
- Research activities
- Written short- and long-term patient management plans
- Quality of life results, post-transplant
- Accommodation and support services available for patients and families

Phase 2: Payor Reviews Completed RFP

If a transplant program meets the minimum clinical criteria for participation as established by the payor, then, typically, it receives notification that it has passed the first screening process, and the second screening process begins.

Phase 3: Payor Conducts Site Visit at Facility to Review Programs and Interview Team Members

Phase 4: Pricing Negotiations

Phase 5: The Facility is Notified if it has been Selected to Participate in the Network

After such a lengthy process, the results for the transplant center often fell short of expectations of increased patient volume. Many payors introduced their new transplant networks via a participating provider listing inclusive of programs considered to be leaders in the field of transplantation. Given the limited number of transplant programs that each payor intended to contract with, it was apparent these networks had the potential to create a highly competitive environment. The key to how competitive this type of contracting might become rested with the payors' ability to channel patients successfully, and in the first few years, many payors and contracted transplant programs found the actual number of referrals through those early networks less than originally anticipated (Koska, 1990).

In hindsight, it is clear that another simultaneous trend contributed to the highly competitive environment for transplant services—that is, the proliferation of transplant programs, which increased in number by 26% nationwide between 1988 and 1990 (see Table 10.2). The combination of increased number of programs, the limitation by payors of the number of programs they would contract with, and their anticipation of greater pricing discounts from contracted programs put great pressure on transplant programs nationwide.

TABLE 10.2 Number of Transplant Programs Nationally

	1988	1990
Heart[1]	120	135
Liver[1]	56	83
Kidney[1]	206	231
Pancreas[1]	29	60
Heart-Lung[1]	27	19
Lung[1]	16	38
BMT[2]	94	120

Sources: [1]Adapted from Hauboldt, R. *Research Report—Cost Implications of Human Organ Transplantation, an Update: 1993.* Milliman and Robertson, Inc. Data compiled from United Network for Organ Sharing (UNOS); published statistics. 1994.

[2]Lutz, S. (1992). Hospitals gird to fight 'disease of the future.' *Modern Healthcare, 22*(49), 22–26, 28–30, 32. Data compiled from International Bone Marrow Transplant Registry.

By 1991, channeling of patients by payors was occurring with increasing frequency. Clinicians and administrators alike struggled within their hospitals and transplant programs to respond to these market demands and to position themselves to compete with other major institutions and transplant programs on a national level through the centers-of-excellence contracting mechanism.

PRICING

It is, perhaps unfortunately, impossible to ignore the economics of transplantation. The impact of the potential dollars expended for transplantation is illustrated by the state of Oregon's 1987 decision to curtail coverage for organ transplantation to expand coverage for basic care, framed dramatically as a trade-off between either providing basic care to 1,500 individuals or organ transplantation to 34 (Welch, 1994).

Estimated charges for transplantation can exceed several hundred thousand dollars and can be upwards of $1 million for a truly catastrophic transplant patient (see Table 10.3). Centers of excellence strive to channel patients to a limited number of transplant programs, thereby demanding a large discount from total billed charges in exchange for both increasing volume and maintaining existing volume. The patient benefits from refer-

TABLE 10.3 Summary of Estimated Charges per Organ Transplantation (1993), for First 5 Years Adjusted for Survival

Organ	Estimated Total Charge
Heart	$252,600
Liver	$364,200
Kidney	$124,900
Pancreas	$70,300
Heart-Lung	$282,800
Lung	$280,400
Bone Marrow	$233,400

Note: Adapted from Hauboldt, R., *Research report: Cost implicaitons of human organ transplantation. An update: 1993.* NY: Milliman & Robertson. Reprinted with permission.

ral to a transplant program that has been credentialed and meets or exceeds established criteria, including survival rates and minimum volumes.

Payors are demanding, and receiving, *"global"* pricing structures, or *case rates,* for transplant services. A global pricing structure consists of a flat rate to include all institutional and professional charges for a defined period of time, which is minimally the inpatient transplant hospitalization. In order to retain a competitive edge, payors may offer additional services as part of the global rate, and/or the transplant program contractor may request additional services. These additional services may include evaluation and a defined period of follow-up care, ranging from a number of months to a year or even for the life of the patient. In addition to the global rate, there may be an additional means of reimbursement for a so-called "outlier" case, that is, one whose charges or length of stay far exceed a typical case.

In seeking this type of global rate, payors are looking for predictability—they want to know, with some degree of certainty, that they will not pay, for example, more than $100,000 for the hospital admission of a patient receiving a heart transplant. This predictability enables the payor to budget and manage its costs and in turn meet employers' demands for controlled increases in premiums. What this means to the transplant programs, however, is that they are potentially being reimbursed the same amount, whether the heart transplant patient is released 10 days post-transplant with only $87,000 in charges, or 50 days post-transplant with $500,000 in charges.

Such aggressive pricing structures require transplant programs to manage care appropriately and reduce costs and, thereby, charges. Cost-containment initiatives in transplant programs currently include the following:

- reviewing appropriateness of patient selection criteria
- assessing home health care utilization to assure that patients are being released from the hospital as soon as medically possible
- exploring the use of less expensive pharmaceuticals
- investigating the possibility of performing the evaluation/procedure on an outpatient rather than an inpatient basis or as part of the transplant admission.

Through continuous and aggressive cost-reduction activities such as these, plus implementation of clinical pathways and superb patient management, transplant programs can remain price-competitive while delivering excellent patient care.

KEYS TO SUCCESS OF TRANSPLANT PROGRAMS

There are several clinical factors that will impact the overall success of transplant programs in the next decade.

Maintaining Adequate Volumes and Survival

A transplant program must maintain adequate volumes and good survival in order to meet the minimum criteria established for contracting purposes. Certainly the decreasing availability of organs has had an impact on volumes, and some programs are finding their participation challenged because of this. In order to better protect a program's participation in a network, particularly if volumes are decreasing, payor education is essential. Programs should employ a variety of methods to alert payors to what is happening with organ distribution in their region and how volumes, and even survival, may be impacted by increased waiting times. For example, if survival rates in a given year fall below expected or previous outcomes, proactive notification to the payors, accompanied by a clinically detailed explanation for the decrease, may protect the program's contracted status from jeopardy.

Securing and Maintaining Contracts

Transplant programs should continue to strive for centers-of-excellence contracts. For programs that already have a number of these programs, there is significant benefit to collaborating with the transplant case managers at each contracted payor to discuss their needs and implementing changes to accommodate those needs. Such partnering efforts can result in increased program referrals. Payors want to refer patients to a program that not only offers the best possible patient care, but that is also easy to work with from an operational standpoint.

Preserving Financial Viability

As medical centers across the nation continue to find ways to cut costs in order to remain price-competitive, financial viability of any transplant program can become imperative to its future success. Few, if any, hospitals will be able to support a program financially that is not successfully covering its costs. Successful programs will continually explore ways to provide optimal patient care at less cost. Communicating such initiatives to payors is critical to their awareness that a program is committed to delivering cost-effective patient care.

Creating Effective Relationships between Transplant Programs and Contractors

The individuals within the medical center who are responsible for the centers-of-excellence contracting for the transplant programs are critical, and often overlooked, members of the transplant team. Successful and enduring contracting can be achieved through a strong working relationship between the contracting managers and key members of the transplant team.

Effective management of this dynamic relationship can be accomplished through identification of a managed care team consisting of transplant team members and the contracting manager. Transplant team membership should include the program medical director, the senior nurse coordinator, the inpatient and outpatient case managers, the social worker, and the hospital service line administrator. This team should be responsible for reporting volume and outcome statistics that payors require, discussing programmatic modifications that must be relayed to payors (i.e., changes in key transplant team members or patient selection criteria), reviewing changes in clinical practices that could financially impact reimbursement (i.e., introduction of new technologies or protocols, or adjustments to existing protocols), resolving operational issues related to managed care, and developing a thorough understanding of the program's marketplace.

Cultivating Effective Relationships with Third-Party Medical Directors and Transplant Case Managers

The more educated a payor is about a particular transplant program, the better positioned the program will be. Of particular importance is the relationship between the medical director of a transplant program and the medical director of each key payor with whom the program has a "centers of excellence" contract. Inviting key medical directors and transplant case managers to spend time within a program—whether it be via continuing medical education or continuing education unit (CME/CEU) courses or a specially designed site visit to review new protocols and discuss emerging technologies—can be extremely valuable in furthering the idea of partnership.

Transplant case managers with the centers of excellence can serve as a major referral source to a program. These individuals often have the first contact with the referring physician to assist her/him in selecting a transplant program that participates in their "centers of excellence" network. Often the "centers of excellence" transplant case managers serve as the patient's link with his/her health plan throughout the course of care.

FUTURE CHALLENGES

As payors continue to refine their centers of excellence networks, many have reconfigured their networks to add additional programs and offer a broader geographic distribution of participating programs, while still others have further limited the number of programs to exact the greatest possible discount. As the centers-of-excellence concept continues to mature, payors are increasingly better able to channel patients to contracted transplant programs through aggressive transplant case management and through financial incentives to the patient in the form of travel/accommodation benefits and co-payment differentials. Some payors offer the patient and her/his caregiver up to $10,000 for travel and accommodations if they use one of the transplant programs in the centers-of-excellence network, and in addition may cover 100% of the charges for a transplant at a contracted program, versus 70% of charges at a noncontracted program.

Transplant programs are feeling the impact of payors' ability to refer patients more effectively and are becoming increasingly more aware of the competitive nature of contracting for these services. Programs must effectively manage costs while implementing technological advances—a daunting task at best. The third-party payors must be thought of as the *customers* of the transplant program and treated as such. This is a fundamental ideological shift for medical centers and their medical staffs and transplant programs in particular. But if the managed care market continues its predicted evolution, given the uncertain impact of health care reform, the well-positioned transplant programs may easily be those that view payors as partners in the delivery of health care.

REFERENCES

Hauboldt, R. (1993). *Research report: Cost implications of human organ transplantation: An update: 1993.* NY: Milliman and Robertson, Inc.

Koska, M. T. (1990). Institutes of quality experience uneven volume. *Hospitals, 64,* 44, 46–48.

Lutz, S. (1992). Hospitals gird to fight "disease of the future." *Modern Healthcare, 22,* 22–26, 28–30, 32.

Taylor, K. (1994). Transplants flourish under managed care. *Hospitals and Health Networks, 68,* 64, 66.

Traska, M. (1989). In search of centers of excellence. *Business and Health, 7,* 11–14, 16.

United Network for Organ Sharing. (1994). Transplant recipient characteristics, 1988–1993. *UNOS Update, 10,* 26–30.

United Network for Organ Sharing. (1994). Transplant recipient characteristics, 1988–1993. *UNOS Update, 10,* 17–33.

Welch, G. (1994). Marrow transplantation, cost effective analysis and setting limits. *Meeting Report.*

PART V

Exploring Alternate Procedures

11

XENOTRANSPLANTATION: BABOON TO HUMAN HEART

Joyce K. Johnston, R.N., B.S.N., C.C.R.N., C.C.T.C.

Human clinical trials of transplantation of organs between members of disparate species, known as xenotransplantation, automatically garner high-profile public and professional interest and scrutiny. Modern communications assure immediate global focus on these intense human dramas, demanding on-the-spot answers to tough philosophical and ethical questions. Long-term survival with xenotransplantation has been elusive. Xenotransplantation nevertheless has become a tantalizing alternative to the conventional transplantation of organs between members of the *same* species, known as allotransplantation, which has been plagued by an insufficient human donor supply. The risk of awaiting heart allotransplantation has now become greater than the risk of the transplant procedure itself; therefore, the operation of xenotransplantation is being considered.

HISTORICAL PERSPECTIVE

The concept of cross-species transplantation has captivated the mind of man for as long as myths have been recorded. Scientific reports on renal heterotransplantation first appeared in 1905, when Princeteau inserted slices of rabbit kidney into a nephrectomy on a child with renal insufficiency. That kidney functioned for 16 days (Princeteau, 1905). There were other reports early in the 20th century, with kidney xenografts having been performed from rabbit, pig, goat, primate, and lamb donors (Reemtsma, 1991). These early experiences involved only isolated clinical case studies; there was no attempt to explore approaches to prolong graft survival or to understand the mechanism of xenograft rejection.

A 40-year hiatus with scientific inactivity followed these early failures. In 1963, Reemtsma and colleagues at Tulane University transplanted a chimpanzee kidney into a uremic patient (Reemtsma, McCracken, Schlegel, & Pearl, 1964). Five other patients followed, with one of these grafts achieving survival of 9 months. Histopathologic examinations of these transplanted kidneys showed the rejection process to be qualitatively similar to that seen in human allografts, although there was considerable variation in the severity of the process from case to case (Reemtsma, 1968).

Hardy and colleagues at the University of Mississippi performed the world's first cardiac xenotransplant in 1964 using a chimpanzee donor (Hardy, Kurrus, & Chavez, 1964). The graft functioned for only 2 hours. Cooley utilized a sheep heart as a donor without meaningful cardiac function in 1968 (Cooley, Hallman, & Bloodwell, 1968). Other attempts by Ross in 1968 (Ross, 1969) and Marion in 1969 (Marion, 1969) were largely unsuccessful. In 1977, Barnard performed two heterotopic transplants utilizing baboon and chimpanzee donor hearts with 5-hour and 4-day graft survivals, respectively (Barnard, 1968; Barnard, Wolpowitz, & Losman, 1977). In 1984, Leonard Bailey at Loma Linda University Medical Center attempted to improve the natural survival pattern of a newborn infant dying of hypoplastic left heart syndrome, replacing her defective heart with that of a juvenile baboon. She lived for 20 days (Bailey, 1985). Her clinical course will be reviewed in the "Case Study" section that follows. In 1991, Czaplicki and colleagues (Czaplicki, Blonska, & Religa, 1992) in Poland placed a pig heart orthotopically in a man. It functioned for 24 hours, at which point the pig heart apparently failed to provide adequate circulation. This protocol utilized conventional immunosuppression and included the circulation of recipient blood through two pig hearts prior to transplantation of the pig donor heart. The encouraging fact regarding this experience was that the pig heart xenograft was reported to be free of hyperacute rejection, a type of rejection described as rapid in onset, humorally mediated, and representing the single most diffuse barrier to xenotransplantation (see Table 11.1).

The struggle for long-term survival of xenografts appears to parallel that facing investigators trying to prolong the lives of allografts before the

TABLE 11.1 Development of Cardiac Xenotransplantation

Date	Researcher	Procedure
1964	Hardy	Chimpanzee to human
1968	Cooley	Sheep to human
1968	Ross	Pig to human
1969	Marion	Chimpanzee to human
1977	Barnard	Baboon/chimpanzee to human
1984	Bailey	Baboon to human
1991	Czaplicki	Pig to human

advent of cyclosporine. The rejection response can be highly variable in both cases. A first step in achieving long-term xenograft survival will be to find an immunosuppressant that allows the recipient to recognize and accept a given xenograft as if it were an allograft or "self" (Deodhar, 1986). The ultimate goal with human recipients is to achieve medicine-free graft tolerance.

XENOTRANSPLANTATION: REJECTION LIMITS GRAFT SURVIVAL

In transplants between closely related species, known as concordant xenografts, the process of rejection qualitatively resembles allograft rejection in that both cellular and humoral immune mechanisms are involved. With transplants between distantly related species, known as discordant xenografts, the rejection response is humorally mediated, generally hyperacute, or a delayed vascular type. The rejection response differs quantitatively depending on the genetic disparity between donor and recipient (Deodhar, 1986). Hence, the level of immunosuppression that must be achieved for prolonged graft survival is greater in the case of xenografts when compared with allografts. Further, xenograft immunosuppression must also be more selective, because the barriers to graft acceptance are greater. Historically, rejection in xenotransplantation has been categorized according to the mechanism that seems to initiate the process, whether preformed natural antibodies against donor tissue are present (as in discordant xenografts) or absent (as in concordant xenografts) (Calne, 1970). This "working premise" is changing as we become more sophisticated in our understanding of the immune response. The human recipient has preexisting xenoreactive natural antibodies that react with donor endothelial cells. Rejection between distantly related species, mainly hyperacute, commonly takes place rapidly; rejection between closely related species is either acute or chronic and may take substantially longer to occur. Because we have not yet achieved long-term xenograft survival, it remains to be seen if other mechanisms for rejection besides preformed antibody, the complement cascade, and endothelial cell activation will come into play when grafts survive beyond the hyperacute rejection period.

In any host, the rejection process is the result of the innate immune system distinguishing "foreign" from "self." Both humorally mediated and cell-mediated arms of the adaptive immune system are accompanied by the nonspecific functions of the innate system involved with every rejection event. The main difference among individual categories of rejection is the immune mechanism that predominates in a given rejection episode (e.g., the humoral mechanism predominates in hyperacute rejection; cellular mechanisms predominate in chronic rejection) (Michler, Chen, & Rose, 1994). Rejection between discordant species is stimulated by the presence of preformed antibodies, primarily IgM, that activate the complement pathway. This cascade causes platelet aggregation, granule release, endothelial damage, thrombus formation, blood vessel ischemia, and subsequent graft death (Cattell & Jamieson, 1974; Jamieson, 1974) (see Table 11.2).

TECHNIQUES TO OVERCOME HYPERACUTE REJECTION

Strategies to overcome the hyperacute barrier to transplant have been targeted at the main mediators of this process: preformed antibody, activation of the complement cascade, and endothelial cell activation. We now know that complement activation can occur in the absence of antibody. Techniques have been developed to deplete recipient natural antibody either by plasma exchange, plasmapheresis, pretransplant donor organ hemoperfusion, or administration of binding compounds (carbohydrates) just prior to transplant. However, the xenoreactive natural antibodies rapidly return to the circulation and may subsequently compromise the graft. Resynthesis of antibody may be partially suppressed by use of cyclosporine, RS–61443 (mycophenolic acid), 15–deoxyspergualin, or splenectomy (Valdivia, Monden, & Gotoh, 1989). RS–61443 and 15–deoxyspergualin suppress B cell antibody production, thereby blocking the action of xenoreactive natural antibodies. The goal is to achieve accommodation that establishes a nonaggressive state between the natural antibodies and complement of the recipient and the donor organ. Complement inhibitors

TABLE 11.2 Xenotransplantation: Rejection Limits Graft Survival

Type of Donor	Mechanism of Rejection	Type/Time of Rejection
Concordant (e.g., baboon to human)	Humoral or cellular	Vascular/possibly hyperacute
Discordant (e.g., pig to human)	Humoral only	Delayed vascular/ hyperactive

have also been studied in an effort to overcome the hyperacute rejection barrier to xenotransplant. One such agent is cobra venom factor, which acts to deplete C3. Another maneuver is to place human inhibitors of complement (proteins) into donor endothelial cells by genetic engineering. These rejection-promoting factors must be depleted or in other ways compromised permanently for the best long-term results. Resting endothelial cells promote anticoagulation and thus maintain normal blood flow; activated endothelial cells promote coagulation and thrombosis. Monoclonal antibodies and techniques that produce peptides that interfere with endothelial cell activation are being developed (Rose, Pepino, & Fuzesi, 1990).

Investigators are looking beyond early graft survival, hoping to encourage later "accommodation" even in the presence of antibody and complement. Accommodation can be conceptualized as a condition of dynamic tension between the donor and recipient of discordant xenografts, in which preformed natural antibodies and perhaps complement are depleted from the recipient for an unspecified time and then allowed to return to the circulation, resulting in continued graft survival despite the presence of donor-reactive antibody. Potential mechanisms to explain this phenomenon include donor graft endothelial cell antigen modulation, resistance of graft endothelial cells to complement activity, and modulation of the binding capabilities of natural antibody (Platt & Bach, 1991).

Many of the immunosuppressive strategies under investigation are directed at cell-mediated rejection (cyclosporine-based immunosuppression, total lymphoid irradiation, and antithymocyte globulin) as well as humorally based rejection (total lymphoid irradiation, methotrexate, RS–61443, splenectomy, and 15–deoxyspergualin). A further therapeutic modality, photochemotherapy, has been developed that targets donor-specific suppression of both humorally mediated and cell-mediated mechanisms of the host immune system (Rose et al., 1990). New, more potent and selective immunosuppressive agents such as FK506, rapamycin, RS–61443, 15–deoxyspergualin, and Brequinar sodium may result in significant prolongation of graft survival after cardiac xenotransplantation while limiting the amount of generalized immunosuppression, thereby reducing infectious sequelae. These strategies represent a first step toward the ultimate goal of developing a state of tolerance that occurs without medication, known as chimerism (see Table 11.3).

NURSING CARE ISSUES AND RESPONSIBILITIES

When primates are used as the donor source, the physical care of recipients varies little from the care of recipients who receive allografts. The nurse retains the role of balancing the many aspects of the transplant process. On the more distant horizon, when graft tolerance becomes a reality, perhaps very little will be done post-transplant except for routine postoperative care, because the threat of rejection will be diminished. The nurse retains her central role in helping transplant recipients get through the transplantation process. Caregivers must deal with the challenges of recognizing rejection and interviewing to ameliorate this process using newer, more potent, more selective, and more sophisticated immunosuppressive drugs. Controlling the side effects of these potent therapies, especially monitoring for infection, becomes paramount. The primary management challenges will include balancing complex interactions in this polypharmaceutical state. An increased awareness and understanding of the mechanism of the activation of the complement system as the triggering mechanism, or one of several triggering mechanisms, in

TABLE 11.3 Intervention: Techniques to Overcome Hyperacute Rejection

Removal of Natural Antibodies with a Goal of Accommodation

- Plasmapheresis (exchange)
- Organ absorption
- Immunotherapy: RS–61443, 15-deoxyspergualin
- Binding of natural antibodies (carbohydrates)
- Splenectomy

Interference with Complement

- Cobra venom factor
- Placement of human inhibitors (proteins) of complement into donor endothelial cells by genetic engineering

Interference with Consequences of Endothelial Cell Activation

- Monoclonal antibodies techniques to produce peptides that block molecular interactions

xenograft rejection, will be necessary to prevent the membrane destruction that occurs with activation of this cascade.

A primary focus of the transplant nurse will be the transfer of information to the recipient and his or her family regarding living with the transplanted organ. Until a state of graft tolerance is achieved, managing the complex interactions of selective immunosuppressants will be an ongoing challenge.

Control of infection will remain an ongoing nursing concern and responsibility. Two issues will be encountered; first will be controlling the usual infectious problems in the post-transplant period. Second will be dealing with the transmission of animal pathogens from the donor. More than 150 infections have been identified that can be transmitted from animals to humans (UNOS, 1993). Only animals raised in captivity and extensively screened for potential infection are used. There will be an additional advantage when using specifically bred-for-transplant donors instead of distantly procured human organs; the amount of potential ischemic injury to the graft will be limited.

DEALING WITH ETHICAL ISSUES

Nurses will be involved in the ethical dilemmas that surround xenotransplantation. With every advance in cardiac xenotransplantation, there will be appropriate and necessary ethical debates. Nurses will participate in the process of informed consent and will guard patient confidentiality. They will be instrumental in patient/family interaction and will help the patient deal with the practical psychological problems of xenotransplantation; for example, how they view themselves and how they respond to other peoples' reactions (Veatch, 1986).

Case Study: Baby Fae

In October 1984, Baby Fae became the first infant to demonstrate that newborns could also benefit from heart replacement therapy. She was born with hypoplastic left heart syndrome, a congenital heart defect characterized as an underdeveloped left ventricle that would not support her life for long once ductal circulation ceased. At the time, there was little if any protocol in place for locating an appropriate human infant donor in the short time between birth and the time of ductal occlusion. During the previous 6 years at Loma Linda University Medical Center (LLUMC), cardiac xenotransplantation had been investigated in a variety of neonatal animals in the surgical research laboratory. This early experience suggested the immunologic immaturity of neonatal hosts (Bailey, 1985). This early laboratory experience was discussed with the family of Baby Fae after she arrived at LLUMC. When Baby Fae's parents wanted to explore the option of xenotransplantation, extensive immunologic testing was conducted between this infant and a panel of six immature female baboons who were regarded as potential donors. Selection of a single donor was based upon a negative lymphocytotoxic crossmatch, evidence of shared tissue antigens between the two species, and diminished cellular reactivity of the host to this donor in the mixed lymphocyte culture. The ABO barrier was breached; the infant was type 0; the baboon was not compatible. This barrier had been successfully crossed on other occasions. After prolonged discussions with the parents, orthotopic xenotransplantation proceeded without incident. Immunosuppression was cyclosporine based with pulsed doses of steroids. Graft function was normal during the first 14 post-transplant days. However, on the 15th postoperative day, graft injury was documented by decreased cardiac function on echocardiography and decreased voltage on EKG. On postoperative days 16 through 20, antithymocyte globulin and azathioprine were added. The neonate died on the 20th postoperative day with progressive signs of low cardiac output.

On autopsy, there was minimal enlargement of the cardiac xenograft; there were hemorrhagic changes in the myocardium. Patchy myocyte necrosis was considered to be a result of ischemia. The endothelial lining of graft vessels was noted to be edematous, thus compromising luminal diameter. Many areas of cardiac necrosis were found to be thrombosed. Hyperacute rejection was not identified. Minimal evidence of cell-mediated graft rejection was present. The infant was ABO mismatched with her donor and could have developed anti-A and/or anti-B hemagglutinating antibodies. Either one of these antibodies, or both of them, may have been absorbed onto endothelial surfaces of the graft microcirculation, causing microcirculatory stasis, that is, microagglutination of red cells in all capillary beds. One could speculate that this resulted in graft anoxia and myocyte necrosis. There were no lymphocytic infiltrations in the explanted graft. Baby Fae responded to the xenograft with the same intensity that she would have been expected to respond to an allograft transplanted across a strong ABO barrier (Bailey, 1985; 1990).

FUTURE PROSPECTS FOR XENOTRANSPLANTATION

Baby Fae heightened the world's awareness about the need for infant donors. Since then, a significant number of human donors have become available; however, as in the case of adults, many infants do not survive the waiting period for an appropriate donor. Since Baby Fae, 176 infants under the age of 6 months have received cardiac allografts at LLUMC. Five-year actuarial survival for this group is 73% and increases to 79% for recipients under the age of 1 month (n = 74) at the time of transplant.

One can only wonder if Baby Fae's legacy would have been different if she had followed these 176 infant allograft recipients down the transplant road instead of preceding them. She so boldly announced to the world that babies could also benefit from this dramatic technology. Her short life was full of promise for what was possible. Could the immature immune status of a newborn infant provide the most favorable milieu for a xenograft? This question remains to be answered.

Continued laboratory experience encourages optimism. At LLUMC in 1993, a juvenile olive baboon who received the heart of a rhesus monkey survived more than 500 days on a FK506/methotrexate immunosuppression protocol. This result encourages ongoing animal research that will enhance the outcome of future human clinical trials. It is not yet certain which animal source represents the best donor source for humans. Baboons have a relatively long gestation time and have single offspring, thus limiting the volume of potential grafts. Of concern is the question of the transmission of retroviruses from baboon to man (Bach, 1993). One also needs to be sensitive to society's reaction to breeding baboons solely for donation purposes. Transplantation with pigs as a donor source holds promise, especially in light of current gene-transfer techniques. In addition, the pig has similar cardiac anatomy and hemodynamic parameters to humans. Dalmasso and Bach have shown that inserting human decay accelerating factor into pig endothelial cells does inhibit human serum from lysing pig endothelial cells (Dalmasso, Vercellotti, Platt, & Bach, 1991). David White and his colleagues at Cambridge have developed a pig strain that expresses human complement inhibitors (White et al., 1992). These exciting molecular biological techniques will allow us to manipulate the endothelial cells, the key players in vascular rejection.

The most promising approach to achieving long-term discordant xenograft survival would probably entail a shift in emphasis away from changing the immune environment of the recipient to the modification of donor tissue. Target antigens, which are recognized by preformed antidonor antibodies, could be modified or removed from donor tissue by techniques of genetic engineering (White, Van der Borgarde, & Lim, 1991). Another approach under consideration has been the use of xenografts as a bridge to allotransplantation, to be used as a stopgap measure until an ideal human donor can be located. However, it is not clear whether the recipient might develop antidonor antibodies that might complicate a subsequent allograft (Cooper, 1992).

Whichever pathway we go down, it is clear that we are looking at additional human clinical trials with animals as the donor source. The question remains: When has there been a sufficient degree of success in the research laboratory that will warrant clinical application? It remains to be seen what clinically urgent situation, devoid of suitable alternative, will be the impetus for this clinical trial.

ACKNOWLEDGMENT

The author wishes to thank Sandra Nehlsen-Cannarella, Ph.D., and Lori J. West, M.D., for their critical reviews in preparation of this manuscript.

REFERENCES

Bach, F. H. (1993). Xenotransplantation: A view to the future. *Transplantation Proceedings, 25,* 25–29.

Bailey, L. L. (1985). Role of cardiac replacement in the neonate. *Heart Transplantation, 4,* 506–509.

Bailey, L. L. (1990). Another look at cardiac xenotransplantation. *Journal of Cardiothoracic Surgery, 5,* 210–218.

Bailey, L. L., Nehlsen-Cannarella, S. L., & Concepcion, W. (1985). Baboon-to-human cardiac xenotransplantation in a neonate. *Journal of the American Medical Association, 254,* 3321–3329.

Barnard, C. N. (1968). A human cardiac transplant: An interim report of a successful operation performed at Groote Schuur Hospital, Capetown. South *African Medical Journal, 41,* 1271–1274.

Barnard, C. N., Wolpowitz, A., & Losman, J. G. (1977). Heterotopic cardiac transplantation with a xenograft for assistance of the left heart in cardiogenic shock after cardiopulmonary bypass. *South African Medical Journal, 52,* 1035–1038.

Calne, R. Y. (1970). Organ transplantation between widely disparate species. *Transplantation Proceedings, 2,* 550.

Cattell, V., & Jamieson, S. W. (1974) Hyperacute rejection of guinea-pig to rat cardiac xenografts. *Journal of Pathology, 115,* 183–189.

Cooley, D. A., Hallman, G. L., & Bloodwell, R. D. (1968). Human heart transplantation: Experience with 12 cases. *American Journal of Cardiology, 22,* 804–810.

Cooper, D. K. C. (1992). Is xenotransplantation a realistic clinical option? *Transplantation Proceedings, 24,* 2393–2396.

Czaplicki, J., Blonska, B., & Religa, Z. (1992). The lack of hyperacute xenogeneic heart transplant rejection in a human. *Journal of Heart Lung Transplantation, 11,* 393–397.

Dalmasso, A. P., Vercellotti, G. M., Platt, J. L., & Bach, F. H. (1991). Inhibition of complement-mediated endothelial cell cytotoxicity by decay accelerating factor: Potential for prevention of xenograft hyperacute rejection. *Transplantation, 52,* 530–533.

Deodhar, S. D. (1986). Review of xenografts in organ transplantation. *Transplantation Proceedings, 18*(Suppl. 1), 83–87.

Hardy, J. D., Kurrus, F. E., & Chavez, C. M. (1964). Heart transplantation in man: Developmental studies and report of a case. *Journal of the American Medical Association, 188,* 114–122

Jamieson, S. W. (1974). Xenograft hyperacute rejection: A new model. *Transplantation, 17,* 533–534.

Marion, P. (1969). Les transplantations cardiaques et les transplantations hepatiques. *Lyon Medicine, 222,* 585.

Michler, R. E., Chen, J. M., & Rose, E. A. (1994). Cardiac xenotransplantation: Insurmountable barrier or clinical reality? *Advances in Cardiac Surgery, 5,* 231–245.

Platt, J. L., & Bach, F. H. (1991). The barrier to xenotransplantation. *Transplantation, 52,* 937–947.

Princeteau, M. (1905). Greffe re'nale. *Journal of Medicine/Bordeaux, 26,* 349.

Reemtsma, K. (1968). Heterotransplantation. In F. Rappaport & J. Dausset (Eds.). *Human transplantation* (pp. 357–366). Orlando, FL: Grune and Stratton.

Reemtsma, K. (1991). Xenotransplantation: A brief history of clinical experiences: 1900–1965. In D. K. C. Cooper, E. Kemp, & K. Reemtsma (Eds.), *Xenotransplantation* (pp. 10–12). New York: Springer-Verlag.

Reemtsma, K., McCracken, B. H., Schlegel, J. U., & Pearl, M. A. (1964). Renal heterotransplantation in man. *Annals of Surgery, 160,* 384–408.

Rose, E. A., Pepino, P., & Fuzesi, L. (1990). Cardiac xenotransplantation. *Progress in Cardiovascular Diseases, 33,* 105–117.

Ross, D. N. (1969). In H. Shapiro (Ed.), *Experience with human heart transplantation* (pp. 227–228). Durban: Butterworths.

United Network for Organ Sharing. (1993). Xenograft recipient dies: Variations in therapy failed to prevent sepsis. *UNOS Update,* 11–12.

Valdivia, L. A., Monden, M., & Gotoh, M. (1989). Prolonged cardiac xenograft survival by 15–deoxyspergualin combined with splenectomy. *Transplantation Proceedings, 21,* 532–533.

Veatch, R. M. (1986). The ethics of xenografts. *Transplantation Proceedings, 18*(Suppl. 2), 93–97.

White, D. J. G., Ogleby, T., Liszewski, M. K., Tedja, I., Hourcade, D., Wang, M-W., Wright, L., Wallwork, J., & Atkinson, J. P. (1992). Expression of human decay accelerating factor or membrane cofactor protein genes on mouse cells. *Transplantation Proceedings, 24,* 474–476.

White, D. J. G., Van der Borgarde, J., & Lim, S. M. L. (1991). The immunology of xenotransplantation. *Annals of the Academy of Medicine, 20,* 770–776.

12

XENOTRANSPLANTATION: BABOON TO HUMAN LIVER

Leslie Siconolfi, R.N., M.S.N., C.C.R.N., C.P.A.N.

At the University of Pittsburgh Medical Center (UPMC) an average of three patients per week die while awaiting liver transplant. During the fall of 1991, the decision was made not to transplant patients with terminal liver disease resulting from Hepatitis B virus (HBV). This was based upon the fact that all recipients transplanted due to HBV were presenting with recurrent development of the virus in their donor organ grafts. The majority of other programs across the country also deny transplant to such patients for the same reason (Dubernard & Flye, 1991). Therefore, other options in lieu of human liver transplant required serious consideration.

Preliminary studies suggest that the baboon liver cannot be infected with HBV (Starzl et al., 1994). The use of baboon livers could potentially save patients from dying. If the grafts proved successful, baboon livers could become part of the solution to the growing organ donor shortage, and perhaps lead toward the accepted use of other animal organs for transplantation. Due to the volatile nature of such advanced concepts, a host of clinical and ethical issues had to be explored regarding plans for such landmark operations.

HISTORICAL PERSPECTIVE

Nationally, more than 32,000 people are awaiting transplant, and eight die each day without receiving a transplant (Center for Organ Recovery & Education, Update Newsletter, March, 1994). By the year 2010, statistics indicate that one of every 20 people will require some type of organ or tissue transplant (Center for Organ Recovery & Education, personal communication, 1994). Thus, the scope of options beyond human organ transplant must be explored. One of those options is xenotransplantation, or animal-to-human organ transplants.

The concept of xenotransplantation is not new. Attempts date as far back as 1900. The majority of these early attempts resulted in total or near-total failure (Dubernard & Flye, 1991). At that time in history, there was a limited knowledge base regarding organ transplantation in general. The concept of organ donation was very new, and immunosuppressive therapy was not yet available. Brain death criteria which would later assist in determining the availability of human organs had not been established. Cardiopulmonary bypass was in its infancy. Established dialysis programs were too few in number to meet the growing patient demand. Many patients succumbed to infections which proved to be deadly because antibiotic therapy was not well defined. In spite of such a notable lack of resources, the original pioneers in the field of xenotransplantation should be commended for having the courage to pursue such an ambitious goal.

Today, the use of animal organs can be viewed more realistically as a treatment option. This is largely due to technological advancements, greater expertise in surgical and vascular technique, the inception of immunosuppressive therapy, and refined infection control practices. Studies continued, next focusing on the use of experimental measures to sustain life pre-transplant. Within the last 10 years noted advancements have been made, as listed in Table 12.1. These advancements have been of paramount importance to the population of patients suffering with liver disease. In 1991, the concept of porcine-to-human cross-circulation, or "liver dialysis," came to the forefront of the transplant world (Howard, 1992). Genetic manipulation of animals and cross-breeding with human genes are being researched as realistic possibilities for the future. Scientists and physicians continue to pursue success in the field of genetics today. And finally, artificial liver systems became available, offering a mechanism to improve the health of a patient prior to transplant, and in some cases allowing damaged livers to heal without requiring transplant at all (Rozga et al., 1993). As a result of these clinical advances, the idea of xenotransplantation was seriously considered once again as an option.

TABLE 12.1 Temporary/Experimental Measures to Sustain Life Prior to Organ Transplantation

Measures to sustain life pretransplant

- Human-to-human cross-circulation
- Charcoal hemoperfusion
- Plasmapheresis
- Animal-to-human cross-circulation, pig model
- Genetic manipulation of animals
- Injection of donor bone marrow
- Living-related organ donation
- Use of artificial organs

Source: Adapted from *Xenotransplantation: The Transplantation of Organs and Tissues Between Species*, by D. K. C. Cooper, E. Kemp, K. Reemtsma, and D. J. G. White (Eds.), 1991. Berlin: Springer-Verlag.

DEFINING GRAFT CLASSIFICATION IN XENOTRANSPLANTATION

The genetic relationship between the donor and the recipient is used currently to classify grafts into four broad groups (Dubernard & Flye, 1991):

- An *autograft* consists of tissue transplanted from one part of the body to another, in the same individual. Grafting skin in burn patients from a healthy site to a damaged area is an example.
- An *isograft* is a transplant between genetically identical individuals, for example, between monozygotic twins, or between members of the same inbred strain of experimental animal.
- An *allograft* is a transplant between genetically nonidentical members of the same species, exemplified by cadaveric organ transplantation.
- A *xenograft* consists of a graft transplanted between members of *different* species, such as a baboon liver transplanted into a human.

Species which are genetically closest to humans are called *concordant*, while those further distant are known as *discordant* species.

CHOICE OF SPECIES FOR LIVER XENOTRANSPLANTATION

The animal closest to a human in the genetic hierarchy is the chimpanzee. Although biologically superior donors, the threat of extinction and export limitations prevent their use. Next in line is the gorilla, but that species is also in danger of extinction. The baboon is third in genetic relation to humans, and is currently the best available option (Starzl et al., 1994). Baboons are available in large supply. Humans do not harbor natural antibodies to baboon antigens, indicating less potential for strong humoral response (Cano, Desco, & Garcia-Barreno, 1990). The baboon liver also shows the ability to take part in creating its own acceptance into the body, and is therefore considered to be concordant (Starzl et al., 1994). Other species such as the pig have been considered as an option for xenotransplant. However, pigs are genetically discordant from humans, and the risk of an acute rejection episode is high (T. E. Starzl, verbal communication, Jan. 1993).

FORMULATING A PROTOCOL FOR XENOTRANSPLANTATION

The following section describes two xenographic transplants that occurred at the University of Pittsburgh Medical Center in June 1992 and January 1993.

Purpose and Methods

Patients with HBV who have been rejected as human liver transplant candidates were selected individually, on a case-by-case basis, to receive a baboon liver. The baboon to human liver transplant provided an opportunity to study the performance of baboon xenografts, as well as the recipient's immunologic response to them using current standard immunosuppressive therapy (Tzakis et al., 1993). Implantation of the baboon liver also provided an opportunity to analyze the potential evolution of heterospecific antibodies, which would indicate the development of chimerism. See Chapter 5, pp. 73–76 for definition (Starzl et al., 1994).

Inclusion Criteria

Patients considered to be potential baboon liver recipients had to meet designated selection criteria, which included the following:

- Age range of 18 to 65 years
- End-stage liver disease resulting from HBV
- Prognosis of 6 months or less
- Competent to establish informed consent

Of all the inclusion criteria, the ability to give informed consent was the most important. The patients selected were given a consent form that clearly stated that failure of the xenograft would most likely result in death because human liver transplant would not be approved as an option. Candidates were also informed that the possibility of a second xenotransplant might be considered as a life-saving intervention. Because of the severity of these criteria, consent by another party was not deemed appropriate. Contraindications for the procedure are listed in Table 12.2.

Cost

All hospital costs for candidate evaluation and preoperative care were paid by conventional insurance. The costs of the transplant procedure and postoperative care were negotiated with insurance carriers, and the difference was absorbed by the UPMC (Starzl, Update Protocol, Pittsburgh Transplant Institute, 1993). The majority of the costs that were not covered included special laboratory and testing procedures. Incorporated into the consent was a statement that the recipient of the xenotransplant would not receive monetary remuneration for agreeing to participate.

IMPLANTATION OF THE BABOON LIVER: TWO-PATIENT EXPERIENCE

Operative Procedure

Transplantation of the baboon liver was accomplished by conventional methods. The patients were first placed on venovenous bypass, and the liver was inserted by piggyback technique (Starzl et al., 1993). Biliary reconstruction was completed with a roux-en-Y choledochojejunostomy,

TABLE 12.2 Contraindications for the Xenotransplant Procedure

- Systemic sepsis
- Extrahepatic malignancy
- Multiple system organ failure
- Unable to give informed consent
- Symptomatic HIV

Source: Adapted from [Protocol for baboon-to-human xenotransplant, including consent to act as a subject in an experimental study.] Unpublished raw data by T. E. Starzl, 1992.

which is a duct-to-duct anastomosis. The surgeons favor this method of biliary reconstruction because it is technically sound and allows access to the bile duct for monitoring of bile status and for cholangiographic exams. Both patients experienced a normal intraoperative course following reperfusion of the baboon livers, and the clinical impression was one of immediate function of the xenografts (Starzl, Update Protocol, Pittsburgh Transplant Institute, 1993).

Immunosuppressive Protocol

A four-drug immunosuppressant protocol that included cyclophosphamide, FK506, prostaglandin, and steroids was employed for both baboon liver recipients. Cyclophosphamide was administered at much lower doses than those used in its conventional employment in chemotherapy. Except for slightly higher doses of FK506 in the first 2 postoperative weeks, all other medication dosages fell within their standard therapeutic ranges (Starzl, Update Protocol, Pittsburgh Transplant Institute, 1993).

Cyclophosphamide doses were adjusted according to white blood cell counts and suspected episodes of vascular rejection. Gastrointestinal and renal function were closely monitored due to the potential for bleeding and toxicity. FK506 was administered as a continuous infusion and, as with all transplant patients, was titrated according to patient response. FK506 is 100 times as potent as cyclosporine. The drug is also postulated to have a contributory effect on regeneration and repair of the liver (Starzl & Demetris, 1990).

Prostaglandin infusion was initiated in conjunction with the other medications. Some potentially positive effects of prostaglandin that have caused surgeons to favor its use at the UPMC include the following (Starzl et al., 1994):

- smooth muscle relaxant effects, which may improve blood flow
- contribution to improved liver function
- reduction of acute risk of FK506 nephrotoxicity

Steroids were used in the same manner that conventional transplant patients receive them, and were administered in a descending dose recycle format.

The primary difference in immunosuppression between the first and second baboon liver recipient was a reduction in dosage and more focus on titration according to patient symptoms. Patient #2 received somewhat less immunosuppressant medication because the rejection episodes that were expected in Patient #1 did not occur. Also, the potential for infection to develop may have been slightly reduced (T. E. Starzl, verbal communication, Jan. 1993).

Infectious Precautions

The danger that baboons may harbor substantial bacterial, parasitic, and viral organisms is very real. Of the numerous recognized nonhuman primate viruses, the majority have not been associated with clinical illness (Starzl et al., 1994). An infectious disease and treatment team was organized to supervise the studies of bacteria, fungi, and viruses for the donors and recipients (Marino, verbal communication, Dec. 1990). Prophylactic antibacterial and antiviral agents were utilized, including ganciclovir, acyclovir, bactrim, and amphotericin (Starzl et al., 1993). Standard antibacterial prophylaxis with ampicillin and cephalosporin was administered for the first 5 postoperative days (Starzl et al., 1993).

Patient #1 resided in a private room in the intensive care unit (ICU) but did not undergo any infection-prevention protocols that differed significantly from universal precautions. However, because Patient #1 incurred several infections that were not anticipated, Patient #2 was placed in a more controlled ICU environment. This was accomplished by installing an in-room hepafilter system and decreasing the number of personnel permitted to enter the room. Patient #1's infectious complications are listed in Table 12.3 (Starzl et al., 1993).

CASE STUDIES

Patient #1

Patient #1 was a 35-year-old white male, with a history of abnormal liver function since 1984. He had experienced recurrent episodes of bleeding from esophageal varices since 1986. In 1987, he was diagnosed with human immunodeficiency virus (HIV). In 1989, he was in a motor vehicle accident, at which time he ruptured his spleen. At the time of splenectomy, macronodular cirrhosis was noted, and a biopsy confirmed chronic active Hepatitis B (Starzl et al., 1993). The patient was admitted to the UPMC in January 1992, displaying a variety of symptoms, including jaundice, spider angiomas, peripheral edema, deteriorating liver function studies, and increasing periods of encephalopathy. At the time of transplant, the patient had lapsed into a Grade III hepatic coma (Starzl et al., 1993) *(see Table 12.4 for stages of hepatic*

TABLE 12.3 Infectious Complications in Patient #1 Following Transplantation of the Baboon Liver

Postsurgical Day	Infection	Organism	Medication Prescribed
7	Wound infection; bacteremia	*Staphylococcus*	Vancomycin with wound debridement
27	Bacteremia	*Staphylococcus*	Vancomycin
29	Esophagitis	*Candida albicans*	Amphotericin
30	Viremia	Cytomegalovirus	Ganciclovir
42	Esophagitis and viremia	Cytomegalovirus	Ganciclovir
55	Bacteremia	*Enterococcus faecalis*	Vancomycin
61	Sepsis	Presumed after iatrogenic complication	Amikacin and Imipenem
68	Sputum	*Aspergillus flavus*	Amphotericin
70	Autopsy	Disseminated *Aspergillus*	

Source: Adapted from "Baboon to Human Liver Transplantation," by T. E. Starzl et al., 1993, *Lancet, 341,* pp. 65–71.

coma). The patient's HIV status was asymptomatic prior to surgery and did not change significantly following the xenotransplant (Starzl et al., in press).

Patient #1 was transplanted with the liver of a 15-year-old male baboon. Liver replacement proceeded smoothly, requiring only 20 units of blood. The patient responded when his name was called within the first hour after admission to the ICU. He was quite coherent and able to communicate normally. His jaundice was gone. He was extubated after only 17 hours, was eating a regular diet, and was walking within 5 days (Starzl et al., 1993).

Patient #1 remained in the ICU for 5 weeks, although his physical condition was stable. Because there was limited ability to predict changes that might occur, the physicians exercised caution prior to allowing discharge to the post-transplant unit. Also, the uncertainty of the patient's potential physical response to the implantation of a baboon liver caused the physicians to be more aggressive than normal with diagnostic testing.

Following discharge from the ICU on postoperative day 28, the patient had an initially stable course. He was eventually readmitted to the ICU due to

TABLE 12.4 Grades of Hepatic Encephalopathy

Grade I	Mild personality changes Inappropriate behavior (sexual innuendo, profanity) Abnormal sleep/wake pattern No asterixis
Grade II	Increased severity of personality changes Periods of excitation/confusion Patient arouses spontaneously Presence of asterixis Loss of sphincter control
Grade III	Patient stuporous Marked confusion and incoherence Arousable with stimulation Noticeable asterixis
Grade IV	Patient comatose Limited response to pain No asterixis; may be areflexic Highest mortality

Source: Adapted from "Liver Transplantation for Acute Hepatic Failure: A Review of Clinical Experience and Management," by S. L. Smith and M. Ciferni, 1993, *American Journal of Critical Care, 2,* pp. 137–144.

episodes of gastrointestinal bleeding and recurring sepsis. There was no evidence of recurrent HBV infection and no overt findings of cellular rejection according to multiple liver biopsies (Starzl et al., in press). The patient's HIV status did not change in the postoperative period. Ongoing infectious complications were significant factors in the first patient's demise. After 70 days, Patient #1 lost his fight. The immediate cause of death as listed on autopsy was intracerebral bleeding secondary to erosion from aspergillus (Starzl et al., 1994).

Modifications for Case #2

There were several modifications prior to performing the second operation. First, the physicians decided to limit the initial length of cyclophosphamide dosing. They did not simply assume that rejection would occur. Immunosuppressant dosages were cautiously adjusted. Second, a decision was made to infuse a donor-specific transfusion of baboon leukocytes prior to transplant in an attempt to desensitize the recipient further against rejection (J. J. Fung, personal communication, June 1992). The third modification was technical and provided external access to biliary drainage for improved visualization without necessitating an invasive procedure. Prophylactic antibiotic regimens and infection-control measures were upgraded. Finally, the number of diagnostic tests and the personnel performing them were reduced to prevent iatrogenic complications.

Patient #2

> The second patient to receive a baboon liver was 60 years old. He was critically ill and extremely debilitated at the time of surgery. It was difficult to obtain consent because of the patient's declining status. His postoperative course was complicated. He never regained total consciousness. He required continuous mechanical ventilation as a result of multiple-organ dysfunction. A second baboon liver transplant was considered, but due to Patient #2's grave condition, the operation was not deemed appropriate. He remained fully dependent on life support and after only 26 days passed away. The cause of death was peritonitis secondary to a leak at the site of biliary reconstruction (Starzl et al., 1994). The leak was small and was not discovered until autopsy.

NURSING CARE AND RESPONSIBILITIES

Caring for such unique patients presented an exciting and somewhat frightening challenge for the nursing staff, yet none of them refused the opportunity to care for the xenotransplant recipients. They were eager to learn and be involved in such a "cutting-edge" opportunity. The nursing care required for these patients was remarkably similar to that given to routine liver transplant cases. It was frustrating at times simply because so much was unknown. There was limited ability to predict what developments might occur because there was no previous comparison available.

Interpretation of Baboon vs. Human Postoperative Test Results

One of the differences in assessment of these patients involved understanding how laboratory tests and postoperative studies would be affected by insertion of a baboon liver into a human body. Therefore, postoperative monitoring of the patient was quite comprehensive. In addition to routine daily liver and renal function studies, some unique testing was also employed. For the first 30 days post-transplant, *arterial ketone body ratios* (AKBR) were obtained. AKBR measures the ability of the mitochondria within liver cells to produce energy and is therefore a determinant of hepatic function (Starzl et al., 1993). *Complement levels* also provided pertinent information about the patient's immune system. The liver is the primary source of complement (CH100) synthesis (Starzl et al., 1994). In its role as a chemical mediator, CH100 activates the process of opsonization, which is a way of coating cells so as to make them more "appealing" or susceptible to phagocytic activity. CH100 levels were also used to diagnose development and severity of and recovery from septic episodes (J. J. Fung, verbal communication, June 1992).

Specific attention was focused upon normal laboratory values that differ significantly between a baboon and a human (Starzl et al., 1993). Those tests included serum albumin, alkaline phosphatase, uric acid, and cholesterol levels. Remarkably, the patient's levels adapted themselves to baboon levels within two weeks, as illustrated by Table 12.5 (Starzl et al., 1993). The baboon liver itself grew from an operative weight of 600 gm until accommodation into space available within the abdominal cavity occurred. The liver weighed approximately 1,555 gm by postoperative day 24 as estimated by computed tomographic (CT) scan (Starzl et al., 1993). This was indeed one of the best indications that the baboon liver was growing and functioning within the patient's body.

Assessment of Body Systems

Physical assessment of the cardiorespiratory system was relatively the same as that required with human transplant recipients. There were, however,

TABLE 12.5 Comparison of Donor and Recipient Laboratory Values in the Immediate Postoperative Period

	Albumin g/L	Total Protein g/L	Cholesterol mmol/L	Alkaline Phosphatase IU/L	Uric Acid mmol/L
Donor Baboon	18	48	103	387	<30
Patient preoperative	20	63	233	158	481
Patient 5 days postop	20	52	116	452	206
Patient 45 days postop	19	40	171	2812	>30

Source: Adapted from "Baboon to Human Liver Transplantation," by T. E. Starzl et al., 1993, *Lancet, 341*, pp. 65–71.

some additional considerations for evaluation of the renal and gastrointestinal systems. Due to changing serum albumin levels as adaptation to the baboon liver occurred, profound fluid shifts developed. Patient #1 presented with noted edema, which caused discomfort and interfered with his mobility during the second postoperative week. Patient #2, who was not mobile, also developed significant edema. Subsequently, both patients were placed on continuous venous-to-venous hemofiltration, which was effective for improvement. In addition, both patients required hemodialysis treatments due to the combination of toxic drugs being administered (Starzl et al., 1993).

Patient #1 experienced bleeding episodes secondary to recurrent infections that affected the gastrointestinal tract mucosa (Starzl et al., 1993). In Patient #2, the nurses focused on visual assessment of bile formation because an external drainage system was placed during surgery for this purpose.

Neurologic status was a continual focus of concern in both patients. Always a challenge in patients with liver disease, ascertaining level of consciousness was even more complicated than usual. This was mostly due to the inability to predict responses to drugs and clinical treatments that were utilized differently than with conventional liver transplant recipients.

Ethical Considerations

The nursing staff was acutely aware of the risks that both patients were taking. The curiosity level was high within the hospital. Staff members from other areas wanted to come into the ICU and "get a look" at the controversial patient. All of the ICU staff were extremely conscious of the need for confidentiality and made an outstanding effort to protect the privacy of the patients and their families. Other patients in the unit and their families were also aware of the unusual circumstances, and the staff strived to avoid the impression that their needs were viewed as any less important than those of the baboon liver recipients.

The xenotransplants became media headlines as soon as the story was released by the surgeons. It was amusing to listen to initial radio reports in the early hours following the first operation, because in many cases broadcasting personnel had to restate the information, as if it was difficult for them to believe. Public interest was high. The transplant clinic received numerous telephone calls from patients waiting for a human donor, requesting information about the possibility of receiving a baboon liver instead. Following the first transplant, there were two occasions in which animal rights activists protested outside the hospital. All these events took their toll on the patients, their families, and the staff.

FUTURE CONSIDERATIONS FOR XENOTRANSPLANTATION

Based upon the results of the first two baboon to human liver transplants, there are several considerations regarding the future of the operation. Attention will continue to focus on the amount of immunosuppression given to recipients. The tendency has been to overmedicate with immunosuppressive agents due to concerns related to rejection. Neither patient succumbed to rejection; however, autopsy indicated that in both baboon livers a form of "incomplete rejection" was taking place (Starzl et al., 1994). The liver tissue was actually infiltrated with tiny droplets of fat. The fat droplets may have resulted from an incomplete rejection process involving the blood component known as complement (T. E. Starzl, verbal communication, Jan. 1993).

Studies will continue to focus on inhibition of the complement cascade in order to prevent humoral (B cell or antibody-mediated) rejection because cellular (T cell) rejection was successfully controlled with immunosuppressant medication. One of the agents being explored to control humoral rejection is an experimental drug called K76, which is a modified form of cobra venom (Starzl et al., 1994). The drug would need to be administered as a continuous infusion, and due to the complement depletion that ensues, therapy is currently limited to a few hours or days (Starzl et al., 1994). The efficacy of K76 will be unknown until human testing can be completed.

Efforts to prevent complement-mediated vascular graft destruction in more genetically distant, or discordant, species such as the pig have been unsuccessful (Starzl et al., 1994). Consequently, the use of genetic engineering to "humanize" the endothelium in discordant species may be necessary before there is hope of clinical success (Starzl et al., 1994). Reportedly, physicians and scientists are actively researching genetic crossbreeding between species in the hope of providing organs that may be successful donors for xenotransplant.

Dr. Thomas Starzl summarized our hope for the future very poignantly when he stated, "Trial and error has been the only way to rise above speculation with any given animal-to-human combination, providing an example that all triumphs in medicine are the forgotten sorrows of past days" (Starzl, 1992). In spite of these very radical and even startling concepts, two patients and their families allowed experiments to become reality, and for that they must not be forgotten. We must hope that many others in the field of transplantation have similar aspirations of forging into the unknown to ultimately achieve success.

REFERENCES

Cano, M. J., Desco, M., & Garcia-Barreno, P. (1990). Normal biochemistry values in baboons (papio C Cinocephalus). *Comprehensive Biochemical Physiology, 96*(B), 647–649.

Cooper, D. K. C., Kemp, E., Reemtsma, K., & White, D. J. G. (Eds.). (1991). *Xenotransplantation: The transplantation of organs and tissues between species.* Berlin: Springer-Verlag.

Dubernard, J. M., & Flye, M. W. (1991). Xenografts. In D. K. C. Cooper, E. Kemp, K. Reemtsma, & D. J. G. White (Eds.), *Xenotransplantation: The transplantation of organs and tissues between species* (pp. 612–633). Berlin: Springer-Verlag.

Howard, T. K. (1992). Artificial support of the failing liver. *Transplantation Science, 2,* 46–49.

Marino, I. R., Tzakis, A. G., Fung, J. J., Todo, S., Doyle, H. R., Manez, R., & Starzl, T. E. (1994). *Liver xenotransplantation.* Unpublished manuscript, University of Pittsburgh School of Medicine and the Veterans Administration Medical Center, Pittsburgh.

Rozga, J., Williams, F., Ro, M., Neuzil, D. F., Giorgio, T. D., Backfish, G., Moscioni, A. D., Hakim, R., & Demetriou, A. A. (1993). Development of a bioartificial liver: Properties and function of a hollow-fiver module inoculated with liver cells. *Hepatology, 17,* 258–264.

Smith, S. L., & Ciferni, M. (1993). Liver transplantation for acute hepatic failure: A review of clinical experience and management. *American Journal of Critical Care, 2,* 137–144.

Starzl, T. E. (1992). [Protocol for baboon to human xenotransplant, including consent to act as a subject in an experimental study]. Unpublished raw data.

Starzl, T. E. (1992). The future of xenotransplantation. *Annals of Surgery, 216*(4).

Starzl, T. E. (1993). [Update protocol]. Unpublished raw data.

Starzl, T. E., & Demetris, A. J. (1990). *Liver transplantation: A 31 year perspective.* Chicago: Year Book Medical Publishers.

Starzl, T. E., Demetris, A. J., Murase, N., Ildstad, S., Ricordi, C., & Trucco, M. (1992). Cell migration, chimerism, and graft acceptance. *Lancet, 339,* 1579–1582.

Starzl, T. E., Fung, J. J., Tzakis, A., Todo, S., Demetris, A. J., Marino, I. R., Doyle, H., Zeevi, A., Warty, V., Michaels, M., Kusne, S., Rudert, W. A., & Trucco, M. (1993). Baboon to human liver transplantation. *Lancet, 341,* 65–71.

Starzl, T. E., Valdivia, L. A., Murase, N., Demetris, A. J., Fontes, P., Rao, A. S., Manez, R., Marino, I. R., Todo, S., Thomson, A. W., & Fung, J. J. (Oct. 1994). The biological basis of and strategies for clinical xenotransplantation. *Immunological Reviews, 141,* 213–244.

Tzakis, A., Fung, J. J., Todo, S., Marino, I., Demetris, A. J., & Starzl, T. E. (1993). *Human liver xenotransplantation.* Unpublished manuscript, Pittsburgh Transplant Institute and the Departments of Surgery & Pathology, University of Pittsburgh Health Science Center, Pittsburgh.

13

LIVING RELATED LOBAR TRANSPLANTATION

Felicia A. Schenkel, R.N., B.S., C.C.T.C., Mark L. Barr, M.D., and Vaughn A. Starnes, M.D.

Pulmonary transplantation has been recognized as a treatment option for patients with end-stage lung disease. However, a major limiting factor in lung transplantation is the availability of suitable donors. Secondary to the difficulties in identifying and maintaining potential lung donors is the fact that approximately 20% of the patients awaiting pulmonary transplant will die prior to the identification of a suitable donor (United Network of Organ Sharing Transplant Registry [UNOS], 1993). While there are increasing efforts to educate the public and the medical community about the need for lung donors, the demand greatly exceeds the supply. According to UNOS, in 1993 there were 475 lung donors for 1,375 potential recipients on the list for pulmonary transplantation. Consequently, the concept was developed for transplanting lobes bilaterally into a recipient utilizing two living related donors. The candidates for this procedure include patients with end-stage lung disease, such as cystic fibrosis, who may not be able to survive the wait for a cadaveric donor or who may no longer be suitable as a recipient after a prolonged period. This chapter describes the development, indications, techniques, and outcomes of the *first* living related bilateral lobar transplantation program.

RECIPIENT CRITERIA AND EVALUATION

Patients referred for living related lobar transplantation must fulfill both the medical and psychosocial criteria for conventional pulmonary transplantation and must be listed with UNOS. All patients evaluated have a decline in physical status with a life expectancy of less than a few months and/or increasing risk with time of developing an absolute contraindication to transplantation. This is suggested by the following:

- Deteriorating pulmonary function
- Increasing hypoxia and/or hypercapnia
- Increasing hospitalizations
- Decreasing ability to perform activities of daily living
- Recurring life-threatening pulmonary complications, such as hemoptysis
- Increasing antibiotic resistance
- Progressive weight loss

All patients must have the emotional and educational ability to undertake a major medical event and its sequelae. Ideally, support structures should be identified prior to transplantation because these people are crucial throughout all the phases of transplant.

Absolute contraindications to pulmonary transplantation include pan-resistant flora. The sputum must be sensitive to antimicrobial therapy, whether single-drug or synergistic combinations. Presence of *Pseudomonas cepacia* is currently an absolute contraindication. Patients must have no other significant end-organ damage other than their pulmonary disease. Creatinine clearance studies are performed to assess renal status, especially in those patients who received repeated courses of aminoglycosides. Liver function testing is obtained to assess hepatic status. Echocardiography assessment of left heart function and severity of right heart dysfunction is performed. Cardiac catheterization may be performed to determine pulmonary artery pressures and/or the presence of coronary disease in the rare older patients and those with cardiac risk factors. Serologic testing, including cytomegalovirus (CMV); Epstein-Barr virus (EBV); hepatitis A, B, and C; toxoplasmosis; VDRL; and HIV is obtained at the time of evaluation. Active viral infection of the respiratory tract is a contraindication. Bacterial infections demonstrated by an increasing white blood cell count, positive cultures, and/or fever are treated prior to transplantation and immunosuppression. At present, lobar transplantation is not an option for patients who have had previous cadaveric pulmonary transplants.

Relative contraindications to pulmonary transplantation include cachexia (weight less than 70% of ideal weight). Patients with a history of major thoracic surgery or pleurodeses are considered on a case-by-case basis. Patients on mechanical ventilation are considered and pancultured to assess for infection pretransplant. Patients with decreased bone density are evaluated and may be placed on prophylactic regimens utilizing agents such as calcifediol. Diabetic patients are considered if their glucoses are controlled by oral hypoglycemic agents or insulin and they have no secondary end-organ disease. "Semi-elective" patients with a history of noncompliance undergo a "probation period" with frequent appointments to keep prior to listing for transplantation. Emergent patients are considered after intense discussions with their primary caregivers. The opinion of the referring team is the most critical when considering many psychosocial issues because many times they have followed these patients chronically from childhood to adulthood. While the transplant team's opinion is important, it is still a snapshot in time, and must be compared with those of the referring physician before a decision is reached.

DONOR EVALUATION

Initially, as per our original institutional review board protocol at the University of Southern California, parents were to be the only donors utilized for living related lobar transplantation. This limited the ability to offer this as an option to patients whose parents were not suitable donors secondary to results of diagnostic testing or age. Living related lobar transplantation is currently being offered to blood relatives extending to cousins.

All potential donors evaluated have the knowledge and desire to pursue the option of donation. Preliminary testing includes ABO compatibility, chest x-rays (to assess for size), and spirometry. Extensive psychosocial assessment is performed by the transplant coordinator, social worker, and team psychiatrist. All patients are interviewed together with the recipient to assess family dynamics and separately to avoid coercion. Many patients undergo evaluation at outlying institutions because recipients are referred from throughout the country. This requires intense communication between the referring institution and transplant center to facilitate the evaluation process for both medical staff and family. Occasionally, multiple donors wish to be evaluated for a given recipient. Preliminary screening allows for a limited number of potential donors to be fully evaluated, thereby decreasing costs. The drawback of evaluating donors at an outlying institution is that this greatly decreases the interaction between that potential donor and the transplant team. Ideally, the evaluation process reveals the interpersonal dynamics of the donor, recipient, and family members.

Potentially suitable donors undergo a thorough medical screening that includes the following:

- Spirometry with arterial blood gas (FVC and FEV_1 >85% predicted and PO_2 >80 mmHg on room air)
- Routine transplant serologies, sputum cultures, and viral screen (respiratory syncytial virus, adenovirus, parainfluenza)
- Electrocardiogram and echocardiogram
- Quantitative ventilation/perfusion scan with differential split and segmental analysis
- High-resolution chest computerized tomography

OPERATIVE PROCEDURES

Donor Surgical Procedure

In bilateral lobar transplantation, one lobe is donated by each of the two donors. The donor's right lower lobe is used to replace the recipient's right lung, and the other donor's left lower lobe is used to replace the recipient's left lung. The two donors enter different operating rooms simultaneously. The two donors and recipient enter different operating rooms simultaneously. Each donor is placed in the lateral position, and a lateral thoracotomy incision is made. Prostaglandin is administered intravenously to dilate the pulmonary vascular bed and titrated to maintain a systolic blood pressure of 90–100 mmHg. The lobe is procured by developing the fissure and mobilizing the artery, vein, and bronchus. Each donor is then partially heparizined and the lobe removed and transferred to a sterile back table for preservation. The pulmonary artery, and alternately the pulmonary vein, is perfused with approximately two liters of modified Collins solution until blanching of the organ is achieved. The lobe is simultaneously ventilated with room air to remove any areas of atelectasis. The bronchus is atraumatically clamped, and the lobe is stored in a cold physiologic solution and transported to the recipient operating room in an ice-filled cooler. The donor is transported to the intensive care unit with an epidural catheter in place.

Recipient Surgical Procedure

At the same time the donor surgery is being performed, the recipient surgery is begun in a third operating room. A pulmonary artery and arterial catheter are placed, and the recipient undergoes induction of anesthesia with single-lumen ventilation. The recipient is positioned supine, and a bilateral submammary incision, also known as a "clamshell incision," is made. Bilateral pneumonectomies are performed on the recipient while on full cardiopulmonary bypass. The chest is irrigated with an antibiotic solution, usually tobramycin, after the lungs are removed. Each of the two lobes is implanted sequentially. Anastomoses of the bronchus, pulmonary vein, and pulmonary artery are performed on each side. Transesophageal echocardiography is performed to evaluate the patency of the pulmonary venous anastomoses. After warming the patient, cardiopulmonary bypass is weaned, and the patient is ventilated via a single-lumen endotracheal tube. The recipient undergoes intraoperative bronchoscopy to evalute the bronchial anastomoses. The patient is then transported to the intensive care unit.

POSTOPERATIVE CARE

Donor Postoperative Care

Both donors are monitored in the intensive care unit for 24 hours before transfer to the step-down unit. Pain management is achieved with a patient-controlled analgesia unit (PCA) via the epidural catheter. Chest tubes are required until any air leak has stopped and the remaining lung completely fills the hemithorax. Oral analgesics are administered upon removal of chest tubes and continued for a short time after discharge.

Recipient Postoperative Care

Low-dose dopamine and dobutamine are used for cardiovascular support as needed. Ventilatory support is continued until weaning parameters suggest that the patient is ready for extubation. Epidural catheters are placed when the patient is ready for extubation and coagulation studies have normalized. Chest tubes remain until the pleural drainage has decreased. The recipient generally stays in the intensive care unit for approximately 1 week prior to transfer to the step-down unit and remains there for 2 to 3 additional weeks. A noninduction immunosuppressive protocol with cyclosporine, azathioprine, and prednisone has been used in all the recipients. Induction therapy with monoclonal or polyclonal antibodies has been avoided due to concern of infection in the cystic fibrosis recipients. Monitoring for rejection and infection is essentially the same as for routine cadaveric double-lung transplantation.

PATIENT DEMOGRAPHICS AT USC

Early experience to date involves 15 patients (mean age 24, range 13 to 36) receiving either a right or left lobe from the biologic parents (seven recipients), brothers (one recipient), sisters (one recipient), father and uncle (one recipient), mother and aunt (one recipient), sister and cousin (one recipient), brother and uncle (one recipient), cousin and brother (one recipient), and sister and brother (one recipient). Each recipient was deteriorating clinically as characterized by a mean FEV_1 of 20% predicted (range 14 to 30%), severe hypoxia (three patients required mechanical ventilation with 100% $F_I O_2$), hypercapnia (mean PCO_2 75 mmHg, range 40 to 150), marked weight loss (average 76% of ideal weight), and increasing antibiotic resistance. (Three patients had *Pseudomonas* sensitive to only one antibiotic, and one recipient had methicillin-resistant *Staphylococcus aureus* (MRSA.) The mean age of the donors was 40 years (range 20 to 55). The mean height of the recipients was 158 cm (range 134 to 175) as compared to the donors' mean height of 170 cm (range 157 to 185).

RECIPIENT OUTCOMES

There have been two deaths out of the 15 patients with an average follow-up of 8 months (range 1 to 23 months). One death occurred on postoperative day one secondary to *Pseudomonas* sepsis and unilateral reperfusion pulmonary edema. The second death was secondary to disseminated aspergillosis. Both deaths occurred in patients mechanically ventilated prior to transplantation. The remaining 13 patients will serve as the cohort for this chapter. All patients are presently New York Heart Association Class I functional status, and all have returned to work or school.

Pulmonary function testing at 6 months in the recipients reveals a mean FVC of 72% (range 56 to 93%), mean FEV_1 of 70% (range 65 to 88%), and mean DLCO/VA 75% (range 56 to 82%). Spirometry generally improves steadily until plateauing at approximately 6 months postoperatively (see Table 13.1).

REJECTION

The overall indidence of rejection was 0.9 episodes per patient month. All episodes of rejection have been mild, and all have responded to an augmentation in steroid treatment. Rejection episodes have been unilateral in all patients. While the total of rejection episodes is too small to make statistical comparisons, an early pattern has been observed regarding the incidence of repeat rejection compared with a cohort of cadaveric lung transplants performed at our institution during the same period (Barr, Cohen, Schenkel, Marboe, & Starnes, 1995). In the living related lung transplant group, 31% of the patients were rejection-free and 61% had only one rejection. Only one patient (8%) had multiple rejection episodes. In contrast, only 11% of the cadaveric group were rejection-free, 44% had one rejection, 45% had multiple rejection episodes, and 50% of the cadaveric group required adjuvant therapy with either total lymphoid irradiation, Cytoxan, or methotrexate.

The average number of HLA matches was 3.2 (range one to six). The average number of mismatches was 2.3 (range zero to five). While the numbers are still small, there has been no correlation with HLA matches or mismatches and rejection episodes.

TABLE 13.1 Serial Pulmonary Function Testing from a Single Double-Lobar Recipient

Date	FVC (Predicted)	FEV_1 (Predicted)
01/29/93	No data, day of operation	
02/12/93	2.06 (56%)	1.61 (54%)
03/13/93	2.11 (61%)	1.71 (58%)
03/23/93	2.24 (61%)	1.71 (58%)
04/30/93	2.45 (67%)	1.95 (66%)
05/21/93	2.44 (67%)	1.82 (62%)
06/15/93	2.59 (71%)	1.94 (66%)
07/06/93	2.80 (77%)	1.89 (62%)
09/14/93	2.98 (82%)	1.91 (65%)

INFECTIONS

Unless performed urgently, patients undergoing living related bilateral lobar transplantation should have sinus surgery preoperatively to decrease postoperative contamination from the sinuses. Emergent or unstable candidates generally undergo the procedure at the time of the first bronchoscopy. All patients should utilize sinus irrigation with an aminoglycoside solution. Both aerosolized and intravenous antibiotics should be given to decrease the risk of sepsis and/or pulmonary infection in the immunocompromised host.

Similar to cystic fibrosis patients undergoing conventional lung transplantation, serious infections have been seen postoperatively. The incidence of infection is 0.19 per patient month. There have been infection episodes with *Pseudomonas* pneumonia (nine), *Staphylococcus* pneumonia (three), disseminated aspergillosis (one), symptomatic CMV (three), *Pseudomonas* sepsis (one), *Legionella* pneumonia (one), candidal bronchitis (one), and aspergillus sinusitis/pneumonia (one).

DONOR OUTCOMES

Other than prolonged air leaks requiring continued chest tube placement, there have been no significant complications in the donors (Cohen et al., 1994). Donor spirometry after right lobectomy decreases approximately 17% in FVC and 17% in FEV_1. Left lobectomy pulmonary function testing reveals an 18% decrease in FVC and a 20% decrease in FEV_1. Mean postoperative stay for the right lower lobe donors is 7.8 days (range 4 to 17). Left lower lobe donor patients had a mean hospital stay of 9.2 days (range 5 to 19). All patients have returned to their previous functional status.

CONCLUSION

Living related lobar transplantation provides donor availability to those who may not be able to survive the wait for a suitable cadaveric donor. There have been no major complications to the donors, and all have returned to their preoperative functional status. Recipients all have excellent pulmonary reserve and functional status. While the benefits of this procedure are evident, there are risks. Although the majority of our patients to date have been mature adults, questions arise as to whether lobar transplantation will provide adequate pulmonary reserve in growing children. Finally, there is always a risk to every operative procedure, including donor lobectomy. Despite this, living related lobar transplantation offers a new therapeutic option for patients with end-stage lung disease.

REFERENCES

Barr M. L., Schenkel, F. A., Cohen, R. G., Chan, K. M., Barberas, R. G., Marboe, C. C., & Starnes, V. A. (1995). Living related lobar transplantation: Recipient outcome and early rejection patterns. *Transplantation Proceedings, 27.*

Cohen, R. G., Barr, M. L., Schenkel, F. A., DeMeester, T. R., Wells, W. J., & Starnes, V. A. (1994). Living-related donor lobectomy for bilateral lobar transplantation in patients with cystic fibrosis. *Annals of Thoracic Surgery, 57,* 1423–1428.

United Network of Organ Sharing Transplant Registry. (1993). Richmond, VA.

14

COMBINED PANCREAS-LIVER-KIDNEY TRANSPLANTATION

Jane A. Waskerwitz, R.N., M.S., and Stuart M. Busse-Henry, B.S.

Successes achieved following transplantation of a single organ for treatment of end-stage disease catalyzed the evolution of multi-organ transplantation to treat conditions resulting in the failure of multiple organs. Simultaneous pancreas-kidney (SPK) transplantations for Type I diabetes mellitus (DM) with associated end-stage renal disease (ESRD) are the most common type of multiple organ transplants performed worldwide. Select candidates with hepatorenal syndrome may be considered for a kidney transplant at the time of orthotopic liver transplantation (OLT) if postoperative restoration of renal function is not predicted. Once excluded for consideration for liver transplantation, Type I diabetics may now be candidates for simultaneous liver-pancreas transplants.

HISTORICAL PERSPECTIVE

In the United States, the first successful kidney transplant was performed in 1954 by a team headed by Dr. Joseph E. Murray at the Peter Bent Brigham Hospital in Boston (Murray, Merrill, & Harrison, 1955). An identical twin donated a kidney to his brother who had ESRD secondary to glomerulonephritis (GN). Success demonstrated that kidney transplantation was technically feasible and could render the recipient dialysis-free. While developments continued in renal transplantation, other organs were attempted. In 1966, the first pancreas transplant was performed by a team headed by Dr. Richard Lellihei at the University of Minnesota in a woman with Type I diabetes (Kelly, Lillehei, Merkel, Idezuki, & Goetz, 1967). It was not, however, until the middle 1980s that successes elevated pancreas transplantation from experimental to therapeutic status. The first successful documentation of hepatorenal transplants was by Margreiter and associates in 1984 (Margreiter et al., 1984). Four patients were transplanted at their center in Austria in 1984 and 1985. Three patients were diagnosed with hepatitis B and one with cirrhosis. All patients had GN as their underlying renal disorder. All patients had normal graft function post-transplant.

CANDIDATE SELECTION CRITERIA

Results of early efforts at pancreatic transplantation were perhaps adversely affected by the acceptance of inappropriate patients whose neurovascular complications were far advanced. Although inclusion criteria remain broad, the selection of appropriate candidates requires a thorough evaluation by an experienced multidisciplinary transplant team (see Table 14.1).

Both types of diabetics are predisposed to complications, but pancreas transplantation is generally reserved for those suffering from Type I. Three types of pancreas transplants have been performed. These include the following:

- Pancreas alone (PA), which is indicated in the absence of diabetic nephropathy
- Pancreas after kidney (PAK)
- Simultaneous pancreas kidney (SPK)

When considering pancreas transplant alone, potential benefits must be weighed against risks related to the surgical procedure and adverse effects of immunosuppression. Rejection is difficult to detect when the pancreas is transplanted alone or in a second operation after the kidney. In both cases, obtaining insurance coverage for the pancreas procedure presents a challenge for financial screeners. In contrast, patients undergoing SPK transplantation require one operation, which is more often a benefit included in insurance coverage. Recipients are exposed to one set of foreign antigens because both organs are obtained from the same donor.

TABLE 14.1 Selection Criteria

Renal Transplantation

- Irreversible (or approaching) end-stage renal disease
- No age criteria (determination based on physiological age)

Simultaneous Renal and Pancreatic Transplantation

- Type I diabetes mellitus with end-stage diabetic nephropathy but free of advanced diabetic neurovascular complications
- Age less than 60 years
- Strong motivation with realistic expectations of the uncertain benefits of a successful pancreas transplant beyond glycemic control

Hepatic Transplantation

- Presence of irreversible liver disease and a life expectancy of less than 12 months with no effective medical or surgical alternatives to transplantation
- Chronic liver disease that has progressed to the point of significant interference with the patient's ability to work or with his/her satisfactory quality of life
- Progression of liver disease that will predictably result in mortality exceeding that of transplantation (75–80% one-year patient survival, 60% five-year survival)

Manifestations of End-Stage Liver Disease

- Progressive jaundice
- Intractable ascites
- Encephalopathy
- Intractable pruritus
- Variceal bleeding (Child's A, B, or C patients)
- Chronic fatigue (e.g., loss of gainful employment)
- Bleeding diathesis or coagulopathy
- Spontaneous bacterial peritonitis
- Recurrent infection (e.g., sclerosing cholangitis)
- Fulminant hepatic failure

Source: Stanford Health Services, Multi-Organ Transplant Center, 1994.

Because rejection is thought to occur in tandem and indicators of renal transplant rejection are known, prompt treatment can be instituted. For these reasons, greatest success has been achieved and the greatest number of SPK transplants performed have been SPK.

The small number of actual reported hepatorenal transplants may be due to the lack of clear criteria for hepatorenal syndrome (HRS). Inclusion criteria are often vague but indications for evaluation are as follows:

- Chronic hepatorenal syndrome
- Metabolic disorders, such as oxalosis
- Drug toxicity

Criteria for HRS are as follows (Wolfgang et al., 1988):

- Presence of severe liver disease
- Absence of primary renal disease
- Acute onset of azotemia
- Relative oliguria with urine output <500ml/24h
- Urinary Na^+ <10mEq/L
- Benign urinary sediment
- No response to volume expansion or correction of "prerenal factors"

EVALUATION PROCESS

Prospective candidates for multiple-organ transplantation are evaluated by a multidisciplinary transplant team including the following:

- Transplant surgeon
- Nephrologist/hepatologist
- Transplant coordinator
- Social worker

A medical history is obtained and physical examination performed. All aspects of transplantation are discussed in great detail, including potential risks and benefits. It is imperative that selected candidates be highly motivated and understand the uncertain benefits of a successful transplant.

Routine screening studies involve a multisystemic assessment (see Table 14.2). The following functions are included:

- Renal function
- Hepatic function
- Infection and cancer surveillance
- Cardiac function
- Pancreatic function

Renal Function

Renal function is assessed if the intended recipient is not yet end-stage and preemptive transplantation is being considered. The appropriate timing of transplantation requires clinical judgement because platelet dysfunction associated with ESRD can be advantageous in preventing thrombosis. One of the most documented complications of liver disease is renal failure, and transplantation is considered when restoration of renal function is not predicted.

Hepatic Function

Timing of transplantation is determined by degree of liver dysfunction as documented by liver function tests. A liver biopsy may be indicated, if not previously performed, to identify the primary disease process. Further laboratory studies can assist in confirming the diagnosis. Results of hepatitis serologies (e.g., B,C) determine the suitability for transplantation. Currently, only a few select centers perform liver transplants on candidates diagnosed with hepatitis B because of concern regarding recurrent active hepatitis.

Infection and Cancer Surveillance

Results of hepatitis serologies obtained guide clinicians when counseling patients with regard to risks related to hepatitis and immunosuppression. Donor and recipient cytomegalovirus (CMV) status is established to determine if prophylactic antiviral agents are indicated postoperatively. Baseline Epstein-Barr (EB) antibody titers may influence immunosuppression choices and the extent to which rejection will be treated because EB virus infections are associated with lymphoma. Infectious diseases, such as an HIV-positive state, would preclude transplantation at most centers. Hypoalbuminemia would warrant delay in SPK transplantation until an adequate state of nutrition existed because of the increased predisposition to infection. Isoniazide therapy may be recommended prior to or following transplantation when a positive tuberculin test is detected. Gynecologic examinations and mammograms, when indicated, are essential to exclude malignancy. Abdominal Magnetic Resonance Imaging (MRI) is performed on liver transplant candidates to assess liver volume and blood flow as well as to rule out malignancy.

Cardiac Function

Because of the high incidence of occult coronary artery disease, a cardiac evaluation focused specifically on uncovering significant coronary artery disease is warranted. Due to the insensitivity of less invasive studies, some centers require coronary angiography for all diabetics 45 years of age and older. Catheterization may also be recommended for younger patients with nonspecific ST-T wave changes on electrocardiogram, a

TABLE 14.2 Stanford Health Services Multi-Organ Transplant Recipient Evaluation

Pancreas/Kidney Transplant Recipient Evaluation

1. Laboratory studies
   - Chemistry profile
   - Coagulations
   - Virology titers
     - Cytomegalovirus (CMV)
     - Epstein-Barr (EBV)
     - Varicella zoster (VZ)
     - Hepatitis B surface antigen (HBsAg) and antibody (HBsAb)
     - Hepatitis C (HCV) antibody
     - Human immunodeficiency virus (HIV) antibody
   - ABO blood typing
   - Human leukocyte antigen (HLA) tissue typing
   - Panel reactive antibody (PRA)
   - Rapid plasma reagin (RPR)
   - C-peptide
2. Electrocardiogram
3. Radiologic studies
   - Chest x-ray
   - Mammogram
4. Purified protein derivation (PPD) test
5. Consultations
   - Cardiology
   - Gynecology

Liver Transplant Recipient Evaluation

1. Laboratory studies
   - Chemistries
   - Complete blood count with platelets
   - Coagulations
   - Virology titers
     - CMV
     - EBV
     - VZ
     - Hepatitis B profile
       (HBsAg, HBsAb, HBcAb, HBeAg, HBeAb, HBV-DNA)
     - Hepatitis A antibody
     - Hepatitis C profile (HCV Ab, HCV-RNA by PCR)
     - HIV antibody
   - ABO blood typing
   - HLA tissue typing
   - PRA
   - RPR
   - Diagnostic studies
     - Alpha-fetoprotein
     - Ceruloplasmin

TABLE 14.2 ***(continued)***

Alpha-1 antitrypsin
Antinuclear antibody (ANA)

2. Cardiac studies
   Electrocardiogram
   Echocardiogram
   Right heart catheterization
3. Radiologic studies
   Chest x-ray
   Magnetic resonance imaging (MRI)
   Mammogram
4. PPD test
5. Consultations
   Cardiology
   Psychiatry
   Anesthesia

Source: Stanford Health Services, Multi-Organ Transplant Center, 1994.

5-year or greater history of smoking, or diabetes of at least 25 years' duration (Manske, Thomas, Wang, & Wilson, 1993). Right heart catheterizations may be performed on liver transplant candidates to assess pressure changes related to volume challenges. Coronary angiography may also be indicated.

Endocrine Function

A C-peptide is obtained to document Type I diabetes. C-peptide is a fragment of amino acids that is cleaved off pro-insulin to become insulin. The C-peptide level can be measured to differentiate the type of diabetes because Type I diabetics have low or no insulin production from the native pancreas.

Additional Considerations

Additional studies/consultations may be recommended as dictated by the individual patient's medical condition. Particular attention is paid to the presence and extent of diabetic complications.

HISTOCOMPATIBILITY

Following completion of the evaluation and acceptance for transplantation, candidates are registered with the United Network for Organ Sharing

(UNOS). Most pancreases are procured local to the transplant center because a limited cold storage time of less than 12 hours is optimal. As with the kidney alone, the pancreas recipient and donor must be ABO-compatible with a negative cytotoxic crossmatch. Pretransplant cytotoxic crossmatching minimizes the risk of hyperacute rejection. In PA and PAK transplants, human leukocyte antigen (HLA) matching enhances chances of graft survival.

As with other transplants, recipient and donor must be a similar or compatible ABO blood type. When patients are sensitized, a negative cytotoxic crossmatch is required. The waiting time for a liver/kidney transplant is based on acuity of illness (see Table 14.3).

CADAVER ORGAN PROCUREMENT

Recent advances in immunosuppression and improvement in surgical techniques in the donor operation have resulted in more demands for extra-renal organs. The in situ technique was first described by Starzl and colleagues in 1984 (Starzl et al., 1984).

An incision is made from the sternal notch to the pubis. Once the round ligament is divided, the triangle ligaments are divided. Care must be taken to identify variations of arterial anatomy. In the past, anatomical variations usually meant the pancreas could not be procured. Now advances in surgical technique, such as anastomosing the replaced right hepatic artery (originating from the superior mesenteric artery rather than the celiac axis) to the splenic artery stump, have allowed this.

Once the arterial supply is identified and dissected out, the portal system is located and freed. The bile duct is isolated and divided. The distal aorta is skeletonized, and umbilical tapes are used as tags for placement of a flushing cannula. The second cannula is placed in the portal vein.

Once all surgical teams (e.g., heart, kidney, etc.) have finished their dissections, heparin is given and the organs are cooled with University of Wisconsin (VIASPAN®) solution. This allows all organs to be cooled

TABLE 14.3 UNOS Liver Status

• Status 1	At home and functioning normally
• Status 2	Continuous medical care
• Status 3	Continuously hospitalized for a minimum of 5 days
• Status 4	ICU, acute and chronic liver failure for a maximum of 7 days
• Status 7	Temporarily inactive

TABLE 14.4 Cold Storage Time

• Kidney	36–48 hours
• Pancreas	24 hours
• Liver	18 hours

Source: Stanford Multi-Organ Transplant Center, Stanford Health Services, 1994.

equally and removed in an organized manner for transplantation (see Figure 14.1). The maximum cold storage time varies with each visceral organ (see Table 14.4).

SURGICAL PROCEDURES

Pancreatic Transplantation

The greatest success has been achieved with transplantation of the whole pancreas preserved in University of Wisconsin (UW) solution. Exocrine secretions are handled by bladder drainage of the pancreas with a duodenal segment (see Figure 14.2). The native pancreas and kidneys are left intact.

Hepatorenal Transplantation

Surgical placement of the liver and kidney allografts is performed during the same procedure, but through separate incision sites. The liver transplant is performed first through a midline anterior abdominal incision. Once the diseased liver has been dissected and is ready for removal, the surgeon will decide if the patient should be placed on veno-veno bypass. If used, it allows decompression of the portal system and lower vena cava. Once the diseased liver is removed, the new liver is sewn in by anastomosing of the vena cava above and below the graft, the portal vein, and the hepatic artery. Once blood flow has been returned, the bile duct is anastomosed either end-to-end to the recipient bile duct or by a Roux-En-Y limb of intestine (Broelsch, 1993). The entire liver transplant procedure lasts 6 to 14 hours (see Figure 14.3).

The second incision is made in the lower abdomen, and the donor kidney is placed in either of the lower quadrants of the abdomen. It is anastomosed end-to-side with the external iliac artery and vein. The native kidneys are left in situ (see Figure 14.4).

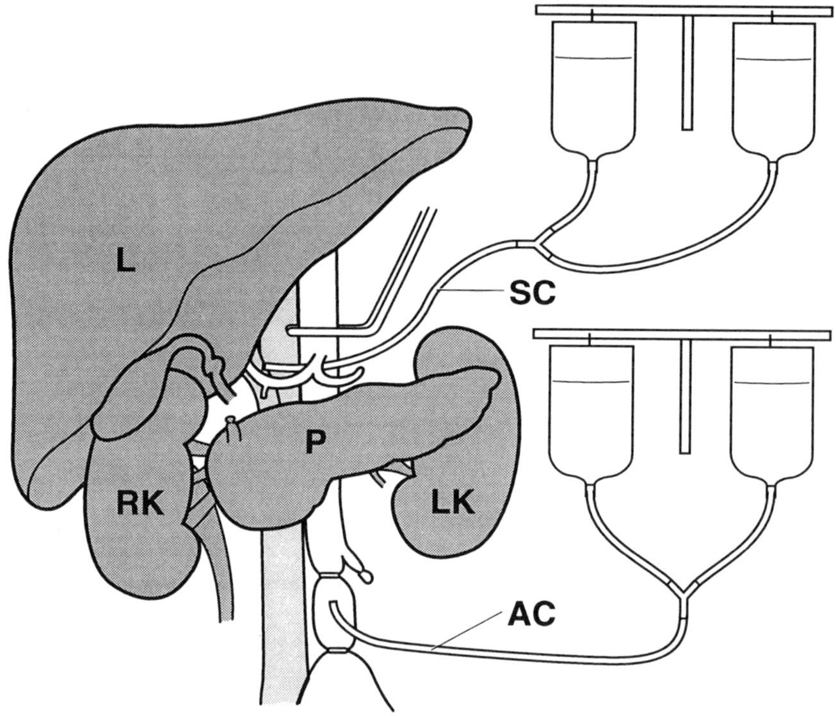

FIGURE 14.1 Organ procurement. Cooling and preservation of donated liver (L), pancreas (P), and kidneys (RK & LK) is accomplished by placement of two flushing cannulas: Aortic flush cannula (AC) into the descending aorta and portal vein flush via the splenic vein cannula (SC).
Note. Adapted from *Organ Procurement, Preservation and Distribution in Transplantation,* 1991. Drawing by Bayard Colyear, Medical Illustrator.

NURSING IMPLICATIONS

Nursing care measures following SPK transplantation can be categorized as those unique to the pancreas, related to the diabetic state, and inherent to transplantation. Following hepatorenal transplantation, nursing care measures focus on the unique functions of the liver (e.g, manufacture clotting factors, metabolize drugs). Routine postoperative care, meticulous observation, and prompt recognition and reporting of signs and symptoms of complications are essential elements of transplant nursing. Responsibilities include the following:

- Administering immunosuppression

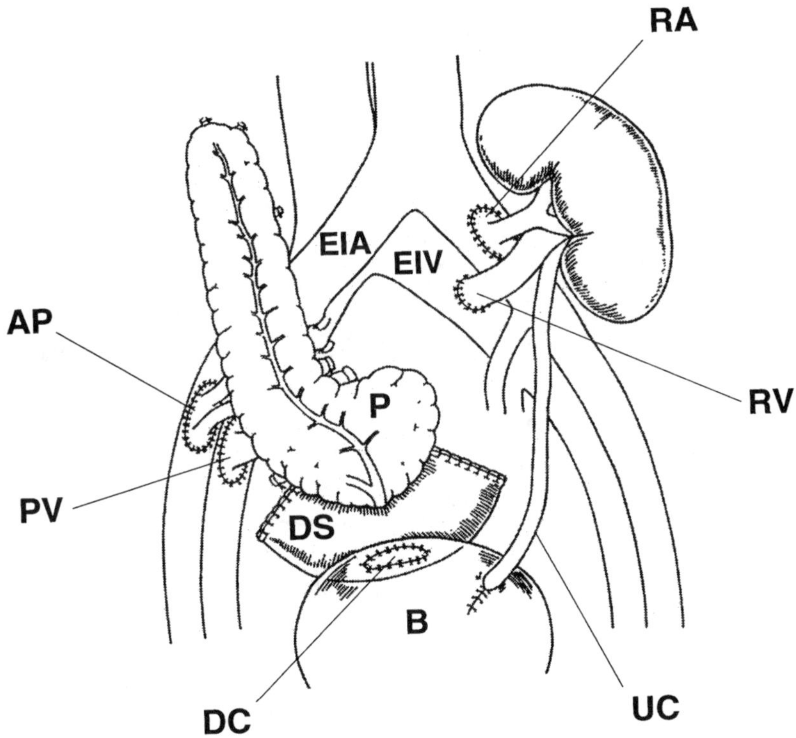

FIGURE 14.2 Simultaneous pancreas-kidney transplant anastomoses. Three in the pancreas: AP = aortic patch of celiac axis and superior mesenteric artery to external iliac artery (EIA), PV = portal vein to external iliac vein (EIV), DC = duodenocystostomy via duodenal segment (DS), which is transplanted with pancreas, providing drainage directly into bladder (B). Three in the kidney: RA = renal artery to EIA. RV = renal vein to EIV. UC = ureter neocystostomy, which allows drainage via donor ureter of donor kidney to native bladder.
Note. Adapted from *Textbook of Surgery* (14th Edition), p. 434. Philadelphia: W. B. Saunders, 1991.

- Monitoring for rejection
- Recognizing thrombosis
- Identifying problems with bladder drainage
- Considering diabetes-related complications

Administering Imunosuppression

Appropriate nursing care measures must be instituted to ensure the safe administration of immunosuppressant therapy, thereby minimizing

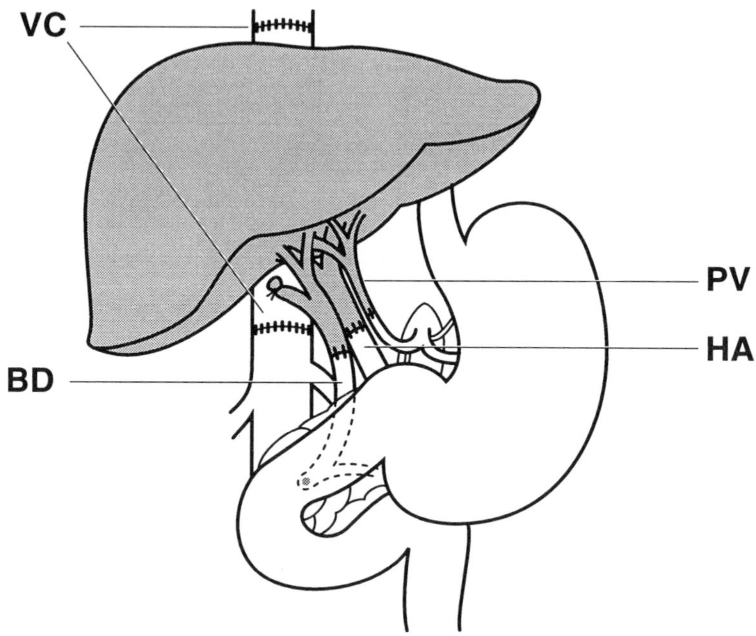

FIGURE 14.3 Liver anastomoses. VC = two vena caval; PV = portal vein; HA = hepatic artery; BD = bile duct, end-to-end; other option is a Roux-En-Y sewing of donor bile duct to intestinal segment.

adverse effects. Triple therapy with corticosteroids, cyclosporine/FK506, and azathioprine is commonly utilized as maintenance immunosuppression for prevention of rejection (see Table 14.5). Because of increased immunogenicity associated with pancreatic transplantation, induction with monoclonal or polyclonal antilymphocyte antibodies (such as OKT3 or ATG) is frequently ordered for a defined period of time (e.g., 14 days) or as determined by renal function. Administration of cyclosporine/FK506 may be deferred in the presence of delayed renal graft function. However, the incidence of acute tubular necrosis following SPK and hepatorenal transplantation is generally low, due to the limited cold storage time.

Monitoring for Rejection

A major barrier to the success of pancreatic transplantation has been identifying early indicators of acute rejection (see Table 14.6). By the time

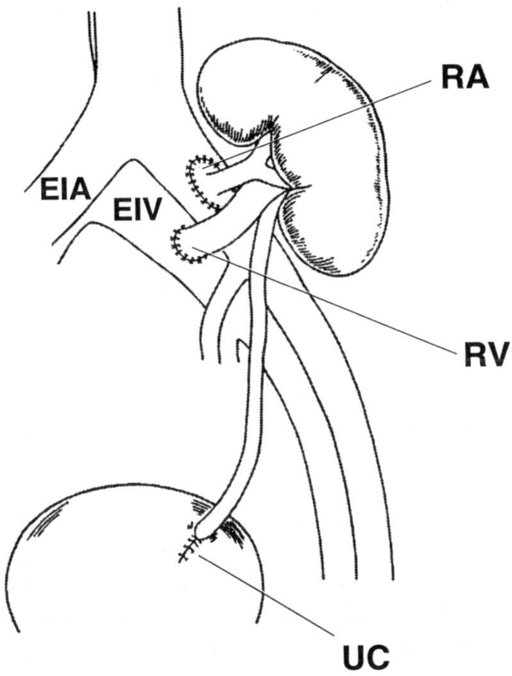

FIGURE 14.4 Kidney anastomoses. RA = renal artery to EIA; RV = renal vein to EIV; UC = uroneocystostomy, which allows drainage via donor ureter of donor kidney to native bladder.

hyperglycemia occurs, damage from rejection may be far advanced. With SPK transplantation, the kidney functions as a beacon by alerting clinicians to the presence of rejection activity. The incidence of renal allograft rejection is relatively low in hepatorenal transplants. Although acute rejection typically occurs 7 to 10 days following transplantation, episodes may be delayed with the administration of prophylactic monoclonal or polyclonal antibodies.

Expeditious treatment of rejection maximizes the likelihood of complete reversal without permanent organ damage. When hyperglycemia (serum glucose greater than 200 mg/dl) occurs, a sliding scale insulin regimen may be prescribed to mitigate against "islet exhaustion" and optimize metabolic homeostasis. Exogenous insulin is otherwise avoided to prevent masking of hyperglycemia. Adjusting treatment modalities is usually effective in reversing rejection. Patients on cyclosporine may be switched to FK506 for rescue treatment. Also, steroids may be restarted at higher levels and "recycled" back to maintenance dosages. If rejection

TABLE 14.5 Summary of Immunosuppressive Therapy

Maintenance
- Corticosteroids
- Azathioprine
- Cyclosporine

Induction Therapy
- Polyclonal antibodies (ATG)
- Monoclonal antibodies (OKT3)

Treatment of Rejection
- Methylprednisolone "pulses"/steroid recycle
- Polyclonal antibodies
- Monoclonal antibodies

Source: Stanford Multi-Organ Transplant Center, Stanford Health Services, 1994.

continues after aggressive treatment, either or both organs may require removal. For liver recipients, emergent liver retransplantation is required.

Chronic rejection occurs later and may be exemplified by a gradual loss of graft function with a rise in fasting and/or postprandial blood glucose. No treatment for chronic rejection is presently available, but removal of these scarred grafts is not always necessary.

Recognizing Thrombosis

Reports of the incidence of thrombosis vary from 6 to 15% following pancreatic transplantation (Dafoe, 1990; Moudry-Munns, Gruessner, & Sutherland, 1994). Acute thrombosis most often occurs within 5 days. Possible causes include technical failure (arterial or venous anastomotic narrowing, kinking, or torsion), disruption of normal blood flow, or initiation of a thrombogenic cascade of events. If prophylactic anticoagulants are prescribed, evidence of bleeding or hematoma formation should be monitored.

Thrombosis should be considered if glucose levels rise or remain greater than 200 mg/dl in the first 48 hours (see Table 14.7). Emergency investigation of blood flow by nuclear medicine scan or angiogram is indicated. If no blood flow is demonstrated, pancreatectomy is performed.

Acute thrombosis of the hepatic artery or portal vein most often occurs within 7 days following liver transplantation. Coagulopathy and elevation of transaminases warrant blood flow studies. Emergent retransplantation is required when the portal vein is thrombosed.

TABLE 14.6 Diagnosing Rejection

Clinical Presentation

Renal Transplant
- Fever, flu-like symptoms (myalgias, fatigue)
- Elevated creatinine, decreased urine output
- Hypertension, weight gain, edema
- Graft tenderness and enlargement

Pancreas Transplant
- Fever, malaise
- Graft tenderness
- Decreased urinary amylase, hyperamylasemia
- Hyperglycemia
- Decrease in glucose disappearance rates on IVGTT*

Liver Transplant
- Fever, malaise
- Elevated liver functions tests, jaundice
- Coagulopathy
- Graft tenderness
- Change in bile color/output
- Tachycardia

Diagnostic Tests
- Ultrasonography of the kidney, pancreas, or liver transplant to rule out obstruction, hydronephrosis, and peritransplant fluid collection and possibly to demonstrate rejection
- Radionuclide flow scans of the kidney, pancreas, or liver transplant to assess blood flow and function
- Kidney, pancreas, or liver transplant biopsy (percutaneous, open, or cystoscopic transduodenal)

Sources: Adapted from Multi-Organ Transplant Center, Stanford Health Services, 1994.
*From "Monitoring of pancreas allograft function with glucose disappearance rate: Calculation and interpretation," by D. S. Elmer, D. K. Hathaway, and A. O. Gaber, 1994. *Journal of Transplant Coordination, 4,* pp. 7–11.

Identifying Problems with Bladder Drainage

Three problems that can occur from bladder drainage of the pancreas are infections, metabolic abnormalities, and technical complications.

Infections

- Urine sterility must be determined prior to transplantation.
- Recurrent urinary tract infections may result from alteration in protective factors such as the bladder wall's mucosal layer, a higher pH from pancreatic secretions, and incomplete bladder emptying and abnormal motility secondary to autonomic neuropathy.

TABLE 14.7 Diagnosing Thrombosis

Clinical Manifestations

Laboratory Findings
- Abrupt hyperglycemia (SPK)
- Metabolic acidosis (SPK)
- Fall in hematocrit
- Thrombocytopenia
- Coagulopathy and elevated transaminases (OLT)

Physical Signs
- Graft enlargement and tenderness
- Ipsilateral leg swelling
- Change in bile output (OLT)
- Change in renal function, e.g., oliguria/anuria (renal)

Diagnostic Tests

- Radionuclide flow scan/angiogram of the transplanted organ to assess blood flow

Sources: Adapted from "Postoperative care" by R. L. Carithers, R. P. Fairman, G. Mendez-Picon, M. P. Posner, A. S. Mills, & K. T. Friedenberg, 1988. In W. C. Maddrey (Ed.), *Transplantation of the liver,* New York: Elsevier Science Publishing; "Kidney transplantation," pp. 81–128, by P. K. Jacobsson & J. L. Cohan, 1991. In B. A. Williams, K. L. Grady, & D. M. Sandiford-Guttenbeil (Eds.), *Organ Transplantation: A manual for nurses,* New York: Springer Publishing; and "Complications of pancreatic transplantation" by D. C. Dafoe, 1990. In L. J. Greenfield (Ed.), *Complications in surgery and trauma* (2nd ed.), Philadelphia: J. B. Lippincott.

- Urethritis may be caused by activated pancreatic enzymes.
- Peritransplant abscesses and gram-negative wound infections may also occur.
- Graft pancreatitis can arise from various sources.

Metabolic Abnormalities

- Metabolic acidosis occurs when the pancreas transplant secretes bicarbonate-rich pancreatic juices into the bladder.
- Oral bicarbonate supplementation and increased hydration are required within a few days following surgery.

Technical Complications

- Leaks may occur between the transplant duodenum and recipient bladder anastamosis and may be associated with rejection.
- Ascites is an indication of a possible leak, which warrants investigation with a low-pressure cystogram and sampling of the ascitic fluid for urea nitrogen content.

- Obstruction from ureteral stenosis at the ureteroneocystostomy and lymphocele formation must also be considered.

Persistent difficulties associated with bladder drainage may necessitate conversion to small bowel drainage.

Considering Diabetes-Related Complications

Diabetic complications can adversely affect the postoperative course of any solid-organ transplant recipient. Ongoing systemic assessment of the multifaceted problems frequently encountered by diabetics is an essential element of nursing care measures.

Cardiovascular

- Cardiac events can occur due to the predisposition of diabetics to coronary artery disease.
- Management of hypertension may be complicated by orthostatic hypotension resulting from autonomic neuropathy.
- Risks of transplant and lower extremity thrombosis are increased by the presence of peripheral vascular disease.

Neurologic

- Decreased vision related to retinopathy necessitates attention to safety and educational creativity.
- Anesthetics, narcotics, and surgical manipulation exacerbate gastroparesis (delayed gastric emptying).
- Anastomotic leaks and infections can result from decreased bladder motility.
- Intraoperatively, patients must be protected from heel ulcer formation due to pressure on heels for several hours. Postoperative ambulation must begin promptly to prevent decubitus ulcer formation induced by immobility.

SURVIVAL RATES

From 1966 to July 31, 1993, 4,891 pancreas transplants have been performed worldwide, as reported by the International Pancreas Transplant Registry (IPTR) (Moudry-Munns et al., 1994). With improved success rates in the middle 1980s, increasing numbers of pancreas transplants were performed at a growing number of transplant centers nationwide. The majority of pancreas transplants has been from cadaveric donors simultaneous with kidney and bladder drainage. From October 1987 to July 1993, patient and pancreas graft one-year survival rates were 91% and 72%, respectively. Those patients with failed grafts were returned to insulin therapy. Although no differences were evident with regard to patient survival, graft-survival rates were higher following SPK transplantation (76%) when compared with PAK (48%) and PA (51%). At select transplant centers in the United States, 1-year SPK graft survival rates of 90% have been reported. HLA compatibility (0–1 DR mismatching) improved results in the PAK and PA groups. Adverse effects on kidney graft survival were not seen with SPK transplantation.

Results of hepatorenal transplants vary according to the etiology of end-stage organ damage. Studies indicate that transplanting any organ with the liver from the same donor protects that organ from rejection. A significant finding was that renal graft rejection was lower. Eighty percent of all renal transplants undergo rejection, whereas only 25% of hepatorenal patients reject. Further studies are needed, but early cases suggest that hepatic transplants induce tolerance and can lead to a form of donor-specific unresponsiveness (Wolfgang et al., 1988). Long-term success rates correlate with those of liver alone. When hepatorenal transplants are performed for metabolic disorders, that disease process is corrected (e.g., oxalosis).

EFFECTS ON DIABETIC COMPLICATIONS

The beneficial impact of glucose control on the progression of diabetic complications has been long debated. A recent report of the Diabetes Control and Complications Trial (Diabetes Control & Complications Research Group, 1993) supports this contention. A successful pancreas transplant provides near normoglycemia with fasting glucose levels of 80 to 90 mg/dl and 2-hour postprandials of 120 to 130 mg/dl. Because diabetic complications are many times established after 15 to 20 years of diabetes, it is not surprising that normalization of glucose does not immediately alter or retard the neurovascular complications. Successful pancreas transplantation can prevent the recurrence of diabetic nephropathy (Bohman et al., 1985); and studies show improvement in peripheral and autonomic neuropathy, microcirculation, retinopathy, and lipid profile (Land & Landgraf, 1987). Repeatedly, studies have demonstrated an improved quality of life and sense of well-being (Corry & Zehr, 1990).

FUTURE OPTIONS

Recent advances in pancreatic transplantation have resulted in improved graft survival rates and decreased morbidity and mortality. Unfortunately, successful pancreatic transplantation cannot reverse damage incurred from diabetic complications. Research efforts continue focusing on a cure for diabetes and treatment that can be instituted prior to multiple systemic adverse effects. When immunosuppression becomes more benign and pancreas transplantation more successful, it would be logical to intervene at the earliest sign of diabetic complications. Other intriguing future options may include transplantation of isolated insulin-producing islet cells or fetal pancreas and the use of biohybrid devices.

Although controversial, experimental and clinical evidence suggests that transplantation of more than one organ can produce a more benign immunologic host response. It is logical to anticipate that a growing number of multiple transplants will be performed in the future. Hepatorenal transplants will remain a mode of treatment for select diseases, especially for metabolic diseases involving both organs.

REFERENCES

Bohman, S. O., Tyden, G., Wilczek, H., Lundgren, G., Jaremko, G., Gunnarsson, R., Ostman, J., & Groth, C. G. (1985). Prevention of kidney graft diabetic nephropathy by pancreas transplantation in diabetics. *Diabetes, 34,* 306–308.

Broelsch, C. E. (1993). *Atlas of liver surgery* (Series II). New York: Churchill Livingstone.

Carithers, R. L., Fairman, R. P., Mendez-Picon, G., Posner, M. P., Mills, A. S., & Friedenberg, K. T. (1988). Postoperative care. In W. C. Maddrey (Ed.), *Transplantation of the liver.* New York: Elsevier Science Publishing.

Corry, R. J., & Zehr, P. (1990). Quality of life in diabetic recipients of kidney transplants is better with the addition of the pancreas. *Clinical Transplantation, 4,* 238–241.

Dafoe, D. C. (1990). Complications of pancreatic transplantation. In L. J. Greenfield (Ed.), *Complications in surgery and trauma* (2nd ed.). Philadelphia: J. B. Lippincott.

Diabetic Control & Complications Trial Research Group. (1993). The effect of intensive treatment of diabetes on the development and progression of long term complications in insulin dependent diabetes mellitus. *New England Journal of Medicine, 329,* 977–986.

Elmer, D. S., Hathaway, D. K., & Garber, A. O. (1994). Monitoring of pancreas allograft function with glucose disappearance rate: Calculation and interpretation. *Journal of Transplant Coordination, 4,* 7–11.

Jacobsson, P. K., & Cohan, J. L. (1991). Kidney transplantation. In B. A. H. Williams, K. L. Grady, & D. M. Sandiford-Guttenbeil (Eds.), *Organ transplantation: A manual for nurses* (pp. 81–128). New York: Springer Publishing.

Kelly, W. D., Lillehei, R. C., Merkel, F. K., Idezuki, Y., & Goetz, F. C. (1967). Allograft transplantation of the pancreas and duodenum along with the kidney in diabetic nephropathy. *Surgery, 61,* 827–837.

Land, W., Landgraf, R., Illner, W. D., Abendroth, D., Kampik, A., Jensen, U., Lenhart, F. P., Burg, D., Hillebrand, G., Castro, L. A., Landgraf-Leurs, M. M. C., Frey, L., Gorkel, M., Schleibner, St., Nusser, J., & Ulbie, M. (Aug. 1987). Clinical pancreatic transplantation using the prolamine duct occlusion technique: The Munich experience. *Transplantation Proceedings,* Suppl. 4, 75–83.

Manske, C. L., Thomas, W., Wang, Y., & Wilson, R. G. (1993). Screening diabetic transplant candidates for coronary artery disease: Identification of a low risk subgroup. *Kidney International, 44,* 617–621.

Margreiter, R., Kramer, R., Huber, C., Stiener, E., Niederwieser, D., Judmaier, G., & Vogel, W. (1984). Combined liver and kidney transplantation. *Lancet, 1,* 1077–1078.

Moudry-Munns, K. C., Gruessner, A., & Sutherland, D. E. R. (1994). Analysis of United States pancreas transplant registry data. *Journal of Transplant Coordination, 4,* 18–22.

Murray, J. E., Merrill, J. P., & Harrison, J. H. (1955). Renal homotransplantation in identical twins. *Surgical Forum, 6,* 432–436.

Starzl, T. E., Hakala, T. R., Shaw, B. W. Jr., Hardesty, R. L., Rosenthal, T. J., Griffith, H. P., Iwatsuki, S., & Bahnson, H. T. (1984). A flexible procedure for multiple cadaveric organ procurement. *Surgery, Gynecology and Obstetrics, 158,* 223–230.

Wolfgang, V., Steiner, E., Kornberger, R., Koller, J., Spielberger, M., Aulitzky, W., Huber, C., Judmaier, G., & Margreiter, R. (1988). Preliminary results with combined hepatorenal allografting. *Transplantation, 45*(2), 491–493.

15

PEDIATRIC INTESTINE TRANSPLANTATION: THE SHORT GUT SOLUTION?

Sarah A. Martin, R.N., M.S., C.C.R.N., C.C.T.C.

With advances in surgical techniques and immunosuppressive therapy, intestine transplantation in isolation and in combination with other abdominal organs is being performed with increased success. The experience of the world's most successful series of intestine, liver-intestine, and multivisceral transplant procedures in children will be described. Indications for intestine transplantation, candidate selection, surgical options, and nursing priorities in the immediate postoperative period will be summarized. Immunosuppressive therapy and associated complications including rejection, infection, and post-transplant lymphoproliferative disease will be described.

The major limiting factor for the intestine candidate is the lack of available organs for transplantation. Four hundred and sixty-eight children are listed for a liver graft and 42 for an intestine graft with the United Network for Organ Sharing (United Network for Organ Sharing [UNOS], 1994). Approximately 33% of pediatric intestine candidates have died while waiting for an appropriate organ donor in Pittsburgh. This high mortality can be attributed to the necessary size-matching of donors to recipients and shortage of pediatric organ donors. Currently in Pittsburgh, 27 children are awaiting an intestine, liver-intestine, or multivisceral graft. To date, 64 patients (34 children) have undergone 36 intestine transplant procedures. Seven children have received an isolated intestine graft, 23 a liver-intestine graft, and six multivisceral grafts. The current experience with the pediatric intestine patients is summarized in Table 15.1.

HISTORY

Lillehei in 1959 reported on the first isolated small bowel graft procedure (Lillehei, Goott, & Miller, 1959). An intestine transplant clinical trial was initiated at The University of Pittsburgh Medical Center/Children's Hospital of Pittsburgh with the availability of tacrolimus (Prograf) in October of 1989. In July 1990, the first pediatric intestine transplant in the current series was performed. Four years after receiving a liver-intestine graft, the child is attending school full-time, enjoys an unrestricted diet, and is growing normally.

FINANCIAL ISSUES

Intestine transplantation is a costly procedure because financial providers often are unwilling to fund this innovative procedure. The required deposit is transplant-center specific. A deposit is required for self-pay patients. Deposit requirements are based on the average costs of evaluation, transplant hospital stay, and 6 months of follow-up care. Current deposit amounts for an isolated intestine transplant are $250,000 for hospital fees and $70,000 for professional fees; hospital charges are $500,000 and professional fees $70,000 for a liver-intestine transplant.

INDICATIONS FOR INTESTINE TRANSPLANTATION

The majority of pediatric intestine candidates have short gut syndrome (SGS). Short gut syndrome is the loss of the absorptive function of the intestine necessitating total parenteral nutrition support because of malabsorption and malnutrition. Each candidate's anatomy is carefully evaluated, as the type of bowel segments remaining, presence of the ileocecal

TABLE 15.1 Current Pediatric Intestine Experience at Children's Hospital of Pittsburgh

Pt	Age	Indications	Transplant Graft	Survival Days Patient	Survival Days Graft	Current Location
1	3.2	Necrotizing Enterocolitis	LITX	> 1376	> 1346	Home
2	4.3	Gastroschisis	LITX	> 1253	> 1223	Home
3	2.8	Intestinal Atresia	LITX	385	385	Died-PTLD, rejection
4	0.6	Intestinal Atresia	LITX	23	23	Died-Sepsis & ? GVHD
5	1.1	Volvulus	LITX	> 994	> 994	Home
6	1.7	Volvulus	LITX	> 954	924	Died-Sepsis
7	2.5	Microvillous Inclusion Disease	ITX	> 912	> 912	Home
8	1.3	Intestinal Atresia	ITX	> 827	774	Graft removed-rejection, PTLD
9	10.2	Pseudo-obstruction	ITX	> 785	> 785	Readmitted
10	1.5	Necrotizing Enterocolitis	ITX	70	70	Died-Bile leak, sepsis, rejection
11	4.2	Gastroschisis	LITX/MVTX	519	462/63	Retransplanted-CR, PTLD; Died-PTLD
12	1.4	Gastroschisis	LITX	29	29	Died-Bile leak, sepsis, HAT
13	0.8	Microvillous Inclusion Disease	LITX	> 648	> 648	Home
14	0.5	Gastroschisis	LITX	> 642	> 642	Home
15	4.5	Pseudo-obstruction	MVTX	> 544	> 544	Home
16	3.6	Necrotizing Enterocolitis	LITX/LITX	107	60/47	Retransplanted-rejection; Died-Rejection
17	0.9	Gastroschisis	LITX	> 502	> 502	Home
18	15.5	Volvulus	LITX	> 481	> 481	Home
19	3.0	Necrotizing Enterocolitis	LITX	26	26	Died-RSV
20	1.7	Gastroschisis	ITX	> 398	27	Died
21	1.8	Multiple Polyposis	MMVTX	> 405	> 405	Home
22	9.6	Volvulus	ITX	> 398	> 398	Home
23	3.6	Volvulus	LITX	> 347	> 347	Home
24	0.8	Jejunal Atresia	LITX	> 341	> 341	Home
25	10.9	Pseudo-obstruction	MVTX	> 340	> 340	Home
26	1.7	Necrotizing Enterocolitis	LITX	30	30	Died-Rejection
27	3.4	Volvulus	LITX	86	86	Died-Iatrogenic
28	1.3	Hirschsprung's Disease	LITX	> 315	> 315	Home
29	9.3	Volvulus	MVTX	198	198	Died-Rejection, PTLD
30	5.3	Volvulus	ITX	> 232	54	Graft Removed-rejection, PTLD
31	8.2	Gastroschisis	ITX	> 262	> 262	Home
32	1.6	Jejunal Atresia	MVTX	58	58	Died-Rejection
33	0.9	Jejunal Atresia	LITX	21	21	Died-Cerebral infarction
34	4.9	Necrotizing Enterocolitis	LITX	>78	>78	Home

LITX = liver intestine graft; ITX = isolated intestine graft; MVTX = multivisceral graft; PTLD = post-transplant lymphoproliterative disease; HAT = hepatic artery thrombosis; RSV = respiratory syncytial virus. *Source:* Adapted from data from Children's Hospital of Pittsburgh, 1994.

valve, and the amount of remaining intestine confirm the diagnosis of SGS. In the neonate, the intestine length is 275 cm as compared to 5 to 6 meters for the adult (Weaver, 1991). The small intestine is composed of three segments: the duodenum, jejunum and ileum. The duodenum receives enzymes important for digestion; the jejunum is the principal absorbing site, as this segment contains villi; and the ileum is the only site for the absorption of vitamin B12 and bile acids. The ileum has a greater propensity to adapt as compared to other small bowel segments. The ileocecal valve controls the flow of chyme and prevents the reflux of colonic bacteria into the small intestine. The large intestine assists with the absorption of water and electrolytes and storage and elimination of wastes. Some children with SGS undergo successful intestinal adaptation depending on the bowel segments and ileocecal valve presence.

The etiologies of SGS can be categorized as the following:

- congenital (gastroschisis, volvulus, intestinal atresia)
- postsurgical (necrotizing enterocolitis, volvulus trauma)
- motility disorders (pseudo-obstruction, Hirschsprung's disease)
- absorptive disorders (microvillous inclusion disease, Hirschsprung's disease)

Congenital Etiologies

These include gastroschisis, volvulus, and intestinal atresia. Gastroschisis is failure of closure of the abdominal wall in utero with a resultant abdominal wall hernia. Gastroschisis occurs in 1:50,000 live births. Fifty percent of babies born with gastroschisis are also premature. Volvulus is an abnormal rotation and fixation of the intestine. The intestine returns to the umbilical cord at around the 10th week of gestation and undergoes a counterclockwise rotation around the axis of the superior mesenteric artery, followed by fixation to the posterior abdominal wall (Wesson, 1991). Gangrene results as the bowel twists onto itself and the superior mesenteric artery is strangulated. Intestinal atresia is an obliteration of the intestinal lumen due to occlusion or total absence. Intestinal atresia results from an in utero vascular catastrophe.

Postsurgical Causes

These include necrotizing enterocolitis (NEC) and trauma. Premature infants are at risk for the development of NEC. NEC consists of diffuse or patchy necrotic areas of the intestine with gut microflora invading the injured mucosa. There have been a handful of referrals in which the child has required massive intestinal resection due to a traumatic event.

Motility Disorders

Although chronic intestinal pseudo-obstruction (CIP) is a rare disorder, a number of children with this disorder have been referred for intestinal evaluation. Children diagnosed with CIP have signs and symptoms of intestinal obstruction without anatomic evidence of a lesion. Usually there is multiple-organ involvement where organ "dysmotility" is present. The disease components can be characterized as either myopathic or neuropathic. Often visceral pain accompanies this disorder, and the children require narcotics.

Absorptive Disorders

Microvillous inclusion disease and Hirschsprung's disease are the most common absorptive disorders for which children have presented for intestinal evaluation. Microvillous inclusion disease is characterized by hypoplastic villous atrophy in which there are abnormalities of the microvillous involution and secretory gland. Hirschsprung's disease is also a disease characterized by disordered motility. With Hirschsprung's, there is most commonly absence of parasympathetic ganglia cells in the distal colon. (The rectosigmoid is the most commonly affected area.) Due to the inability to make peristaltic waves, with extensive disease the child may be a candidate for intestine transplant surgery.

CANDIDATE EVALUATION

The evaluation process is tailored for each candidate. All contraindications are relative and include the child's weighing less than 10 kg, other major organ-system abnormalities, mechanical ventilation requirement, and sepsis. Early in the evaluation process, a thorough history and physical exam are performed.

Biochemical tests include the following:

- blood chemistries
- complete blood count
- viral titers (including Epstein-Barr virus and cytomegalovirus serologies)

- tissue typing and percentage reactive antibody (PRA)
- tumor markers (alpha-fetoprotein and chorionic embryonic antigen) to exclude incidental tumor.

Radiologic Testing

An abdominal ultrasound is done to ascertain patency of vessels (inferior vena cava, portal vein), and a great vessel ultrasound is performed due to the usual histories of multiple central line insertion sites and need to verify great vessel patency for postoperative line access and urgency of transplant. An upper GI with small bowel follow-through is done to determine the length of the remaining intestine. Liver biopsy findings are reviewed if available. A liver biopsy may be obtained if the extent of liver damage is unclear or to verify evidence of fibrosis or cirrhosis. Evidence of portal hypertension, including ascites, splenomegaly, and presence of esophageal varices, is a clinical indicator for inclusion of the liver in the transplanted graft.

One of the most important aspects of the evaluation process is family education. The patient and family meet members of the transplant team and familiarize themselves with the transplant process through interacting with intestine recipients and their families. Family/patient education is a major component of the evaluation process. For each candidate family, the risks/complications, current survival data, and age-appropriate child preparation is initiated.

PRETRANSPLANT CANDIDATE LISTING

For patients to secure organs for a liver-intestine graft, the patient must be placed on the liver and intestine waiting list. Multivisceral candidates are placed on the liver, intestine, and pancreas list. (If the stomach and intestine are transplanted the pancreas must be transplanted due to vascular anatomy.) The UNOS intestine list is a two-tier system. Status 1 candidates have liver dysfunction and line access problems (no access through the subclavian, jugular, or femoral veins). Status 2 candidates have no liver dysfunction and have line access available in standard sites.

The UNOS liver list is a four-tier system. Status 1 patients require a liver transplant but are stable and do not require active medical intervention. Status 2 patients are at home and require active medical intervention for their liver disease. Status 3 patients require hospitalization for liver dysfunction. Status 4 require intensive care and meet one of the following criteria: They require mechanical ventilation, are receiving vasopressors for blood pressure support, have a prothrombin time of 25 seconds that is increasing, are experiencing primary nonfunction post-transplant, have grade III or IV encephalopathy, and require dialysis or are experiencing uncontrollable variceal bleeding. Due to the poor outcomes in transplanted status 4 liver-intestine patients, candidates requiring intensive care are not considered active candidates.

DONOR PROCUREMENT PROCEDURE

No specific donor organ criteria have been established for the intestine, and liver criteria are utilized when evaluating a potential intestine donor. The ideal donor has the same blood type, weighs within 10% of the recipient's body weight, and is of similar age of the recipient. Surgeons from our transplant center have gone on all organ recoveries for intestine grafts and have had the opportunity to evaluate the graft prior to returning to the transplant center. Recovered organs are preserved with University of Wisconsin solution. According to Funovits, Altieri, Kovalak, and Staschak-Chicko (1993), the longest cold ischemia time has been 10½ hours.

THE OPERATIVE PROCEDURE

The intestine transplant procedure is both tedious and dangerous. Average operating times have been upwards of 12 hours. The liver-intestine, isolated intestine, and multivisceral grafts are depicted in Figures 15.1, 15.2, and 15.3. The liver-intestine procedure involves four phases: dissection and removal of the diseased organs, vascular anastomoses, bile duct anastomoses, and enteric connections.

Initially the liver is devascularized by ligating the hepatic arterial branches and the common bile duct, exposing the portal vein from the confluence to the bifurcation (Reyes, Tzakis, Todo, Nour, & Starzl, 1993). The liver is removed, and a temporary portal caval shunt is performed (Reyes et al., 1993; Tzakis et al., 1993). The vascular anastomoses are like a liver transplant, except the portal vein is already attached to the celiac axis. After the vascular anastomoses are complete, the organs are reperfused. A biliary reconstruction is performed with a Roux-En-Y choledochojejunostomy (Reyes et al., 1993). Intestinal anastomoses (proximal and distal enteric) are determined by the intestinal segment transplanted. The isolated intestine procedure involves vascular and visceral anastomoses.

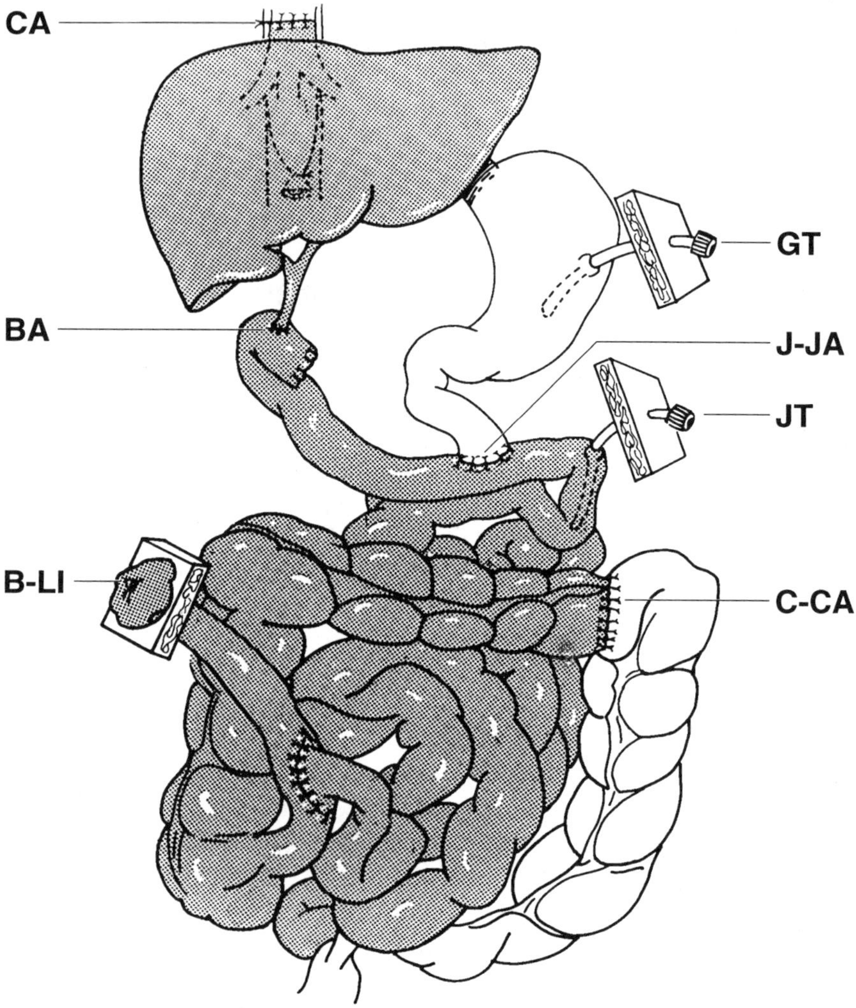

FIGURE 15.1 Liver-intestine graft. The procedure includes two liver anastomoses, two intestinal anastomoses, two tubes, and one stoma. CA = Caval anastomosis; BA = Biliary anastomosis (a Roux-En-Y end-to-side sewn to duodenal segment); J-JA = Jejuno-jejunostomy anastomoses; C-CA = Colo-colostomy anastomosis; GT = Gastrostomy tube; JT = Jejunostomy tube; B-LI = Bishop-loop ileostomy.

Vascular anastomoses attach the superior mesenteric vein (SMV) to the portal vein or recipient SMV. The visceral anastomoses are patient-dependent and may include connecting the duodenum to the colon. Multivisceral grafts have included the stomach, small intestine, large intestine,

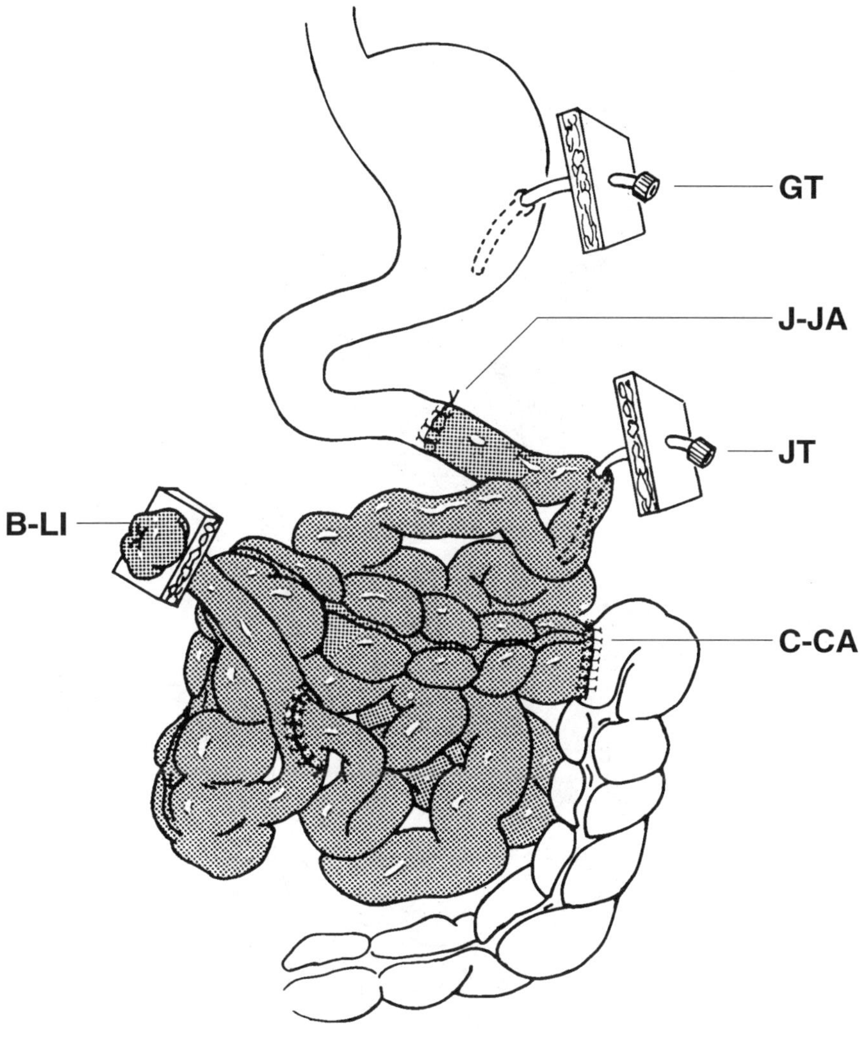

FIGURE 15.2 Isolated intestine graft. The procedure includes two anastomoses, two tubes, and one ostomy. J-JA = Jejuno-jejunostomy anastomosis; C-CA = Colo-colostomy anastomosis; GT = Gastrostomy tube; JT = Jejunostomy tube; B-LI = Bishop-loop ileostomy.

pancreas, and liver. The liver has been excluded in one procedure. The arterialization is performed using a Carrel patch containing the celiac and superior mesenteric arteries (with or without an aortic conduit). Visceral anastomoses have been patient-specific to remaining normal native bowel and can be from the esophagus to colon or endorectal pull through.

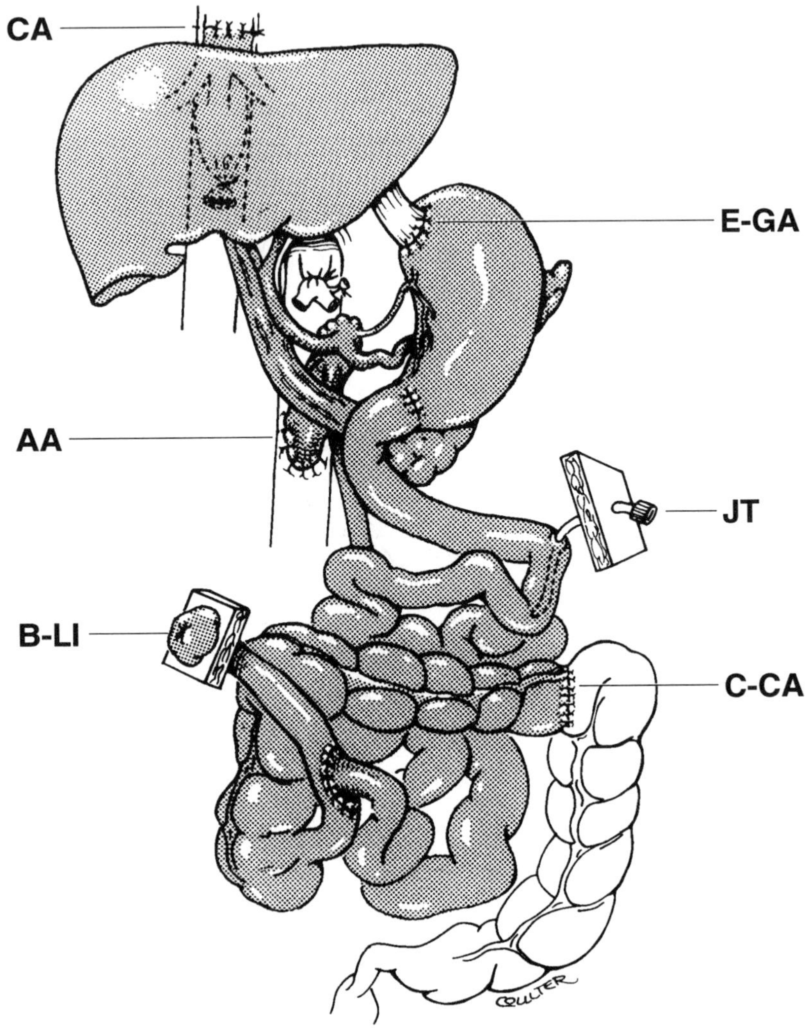

FIGURE 15.3 Multivisceral graft. The procedure includes four anastomoses, one tube, and one stoma. CA = Caval anastomosis; AA = Aortic anastomosis; E-GA = Esophago-gastrostomy anastomosis; C-CA = Colo-colostomy anastomosis; JT = Jejunostomy tube; B-LI = Bishop-loop ileostomy.

IMMEDIATE POSTOPERATIVE CARE

The liver-intestine ABCs in the pediatric intensive care unit include aeration, bowel integrity, and caloric requirements (Cipriani & Martin, 1994).

As with any patient, airway management is the first priority. Bowel integrity is initially assessed by physical appearance of the stoma and enteric output. Normal stoma mucosa is pink, like the inside of the mouth. Initially, caloric requirements are met with total parenteral nutrition (TPN). Enteral feedings are initiated as soon as tolerated by the patient.

Critical care goals are aimed at achieving systems stability with the patient free of a mechanical ventilation requirement and hemodynamically stable. Airway clearance is ineffective because of the lengthy abdominal surgical procedure, visceral edema, and postoperative pain. With the resolution of postoperative coagulopathies, aggressive chest physiotherapy is initiated. Intestine recipients generally require mechanical ventilation longer than isolated liver recipients, due to their overall compromised pretransplant health and precarious fluid balance. Pleural effusions are common, and diuretic therapy and drainage catheters are placed as appropriate.

The enterostomal therapist is consulted because each child has an ostomy (usually ileostomy) and jejunostomy tube (JT). The JT is initially used for bowel decompression and initiation of enteral feedings. The ileostomy allows for assessment of the transplanted graft because the mucosa can be visually inspected and drainage easily assessed. Drainage is assessed for color, consistency, and amount. Bowel elimination is initially ineffective because of the lengthy abdominal surgical procedure. The function of the intestinal graft has been described (Reyes et al., 1993, pp. 289–300) as recovering in three phases as follows:

- Phase 1 is from perfusion of graft to stomal output. Average stomal output for a child is 40 to 60 cc/kg/day.
- Phase 2 is achieved with recovery of intestinal motility.
- Phase 3 is characterized by weaning from TPN. TPN is weaned once enteral intake reaches 50% of nutritional intake.

Enteral feedings are initiated through the jejunostomy tube because the jejunum is the principal absorption site (contains villi) in the intestine. Initial formula strategies are based on donor age and patient readiness. Pregestimil® is utilized when the donor is less than one year old. Peptamen® is the formula choice for recipients receiving organs from donors older than one year. Initially the formulas are started at 1/4 to 1/2 reduced strength with a maximum rate of 50 cc/hr. Peptamen is of low osmolality that prevents hyperosmolar diarrhea. The medium chain triglycerides (MCT) are absorbed directly without the need for lymphatics because they are not transplanted. The patient's oral diet is advanced as tolerated. There are no dietary restrictions. Food aversions have been observed. This is especially problematic for children who have not eaten solids prior to transplant. Peer interactions and role modeling from family members has been an effective strategy to promote oral intake.

Immunosuppressive Strategies

The immunosuppressive protocol for the intestine recipients continues to evolve. The current immunosuppressive strategy includes combination therapy (Prograf, Imuran, and steroids) to maximize the therapeutic benefits while minimizing toxicities of the immunosuppressive agents. Table 15.2 summarizes the current immunosuppression protocol for the intestine recipient.

Rejection

When multiple organs are transplanted, they can reject independently of each other. According to Abu-Elmagd et al. (1994), the incidence of rejection for the intestine recipient is 95% with the diagnosis confirmed with histology in 77% of these cases. Signs and symptoms of intestinal graft rejection include a pale or dusky stoma, an increase or decrease in enteric output, abdominal pain, guaiac-positive output, and fever related to translocation. Routine endoscopic examinations of the transplanted bowel are made through the child's stoma on a routine basis in the post-transplant period. Endoscopic findings indicating rejection include the intestine's losing its fine velvety appearance and possibly initially becoming dusky or ischemic with focal ulcerations (Reyes, Todo et al., 1994). With severe rejection, the bowel may have increased erythema, friability, and ulcerations. Translocation may occur with rejection of the bowel. With rejection, the intestinal wall weakens and organisms usually contained within the bowel may seep out and enter the patient's bloodstream. Therefore, for the first 4 to 6 weeks after transplant and when rejection episodes occur, an admixture of MUDD (Nystatin, Gentamicin, Colistin) is administered into the gastrointestinal tract to minimize bacterial overgrowth. The MUDD mixture is usually a large volume and can be administered as a continuous infusion. When translocation occurs, the patients require organism-specific therapy. This is one of the rare occasions in organ transplantation in which immunosuppression is augmented in the face of a serious infection.

Infectious Complications

Viral infection is the most threatening infection for the intestine recipient. The most common infecting organisms are cytomegalovirus (CMV) and

TABLE 15.2 Immunosuppressive Drug Regimen at Children's Hospital of Pittsburgh

Drug	Action	Dosing	Side Effects	Nursing Implications
Prograf	Blocks interleukin-2 and other lymphokines which promote T-lymphocyte production	I.V.: 0.1–0.15 mg/Kg/dose P.O.: 0.075 mg/Kg/day	Hypertension Hyperkalemia Hyperglycemia Renal impairment Headache Insomnia GI symptoms Hypesthesia Tremor	Side effects greater when administered I.V. Monitor drug levels (1–1.5 ng/ml) Monitor renal function Monitor BP Administration: I.V. continuous infusion oral dosing B.I.D. Available in 1 and 5 mg capsules Don't administer with alkaline substances
Imuran	Prevents cell division, limits the production of T-cells	I.V./P.O.: 0.5–1 mg/Kg/day	Bone marrow suppression GI symptoms Pancreatitis	Monitor WBC, amylase
Steroids	Inhibits interleukin-1 and 2 with a decrease in lymphocytes, including cytotoxic T-cells	Intraoperative: 1 gram Solu-Cortef I.V.: 100 mg Solu-Medrol daily, with dose tapered to 10 mg daily over 5 days P.O.: Prednisone (patient-specific dosing)	Fluid retention Increased appetite Mood changes Hyperglycemia	Monitor weight Monitor BP Administer with food Use antacids Avoid sudden discontinuation Administration: Compatible with dextrose and saline Administer over 30 minutes

Source: Adapted from data from Children's Hospital of Pittsburgh, 1994.

Epstein-Barr virus (EBV) infection. The donor-recipient serology relationship is important because prophylactic therapy is initiated based on viral titers. Primary infections are usually more serious and occur when the recipient has had no previous exposure to the virus and becomes infected in the post-transplant period. A secondary infection is reactivation of a previous latent virus. For the isolated intestine recipient, efforts are made to match the recipient and donor CMV status. Approximately half the pediatric patients have serologic evidence of EBV infection. The EBV is thought to play a major role in the development of post-transplant lymphoproliferative disease (PTLD).

PTLD is one of the most underrated complications of immunosuppression. Twenty-eight percent of the intestine recipients have been diagnosed with PTLD (Reyes, Tzakis, et al. 1994). PTLD is the development of continually proliferating B-lymphocytes, presumably under the influence of EBV. Diagnosis is made by clinical exam and histologic review. Clinical symptoms include fever, lymphadenopathy, gastrointestinal symptoms, and weight loss. Pathology reviews a biopsy specimen. Treatment is controversial and includes holding or reducing immunosuppression and initiating intravenous antiviral therapy (ganciclovir or acyclovir). Ganciclovir is dosed at 5 mg/kg/dose every 12 hours. No pharmacokinetic testing has been done in pediatric patients. Dose adjustments need to be made in cases of renal insufficiency. Nursing implications include assessment of renal function and monitoring for other side effects (neutropenia, leukopenia, thrombocytopenia, nausea, and mental status changes). Acyclovir is dosed at 500 mg/m^2/dose every 8 hours. Renal function must be carefully monitored when administering acyclovir.

Patients with a head-and-neck lymphadenopathic presentation or an isolated single-organ presentation have better outcomes as compared to patients with a disseminated disease. PTLD is a difficult complication to treat for the intestine recipient because rejection ensues with withdrawal of immunosuppression. Therefore, careful titration of the immunosuppression is imperative to promote recovery.

CONCLUSION

The history of this innovative procedure continues to unfold. Young pioneers are continuing to challenge transplant teams to assist them with overcoming the hurdles they face when becoming intestine transplant recipients. The current survival rate for the pediatric intestine recipient is 64%. New therapies are being considered to increase patient survival. The infusion of donor bone marrow to increase patient immunologic tolerance of the transplanted graft is currently undergoing institutional review board evaluation.

Many of the patients are off enteral and parenteral nutrition and are thriving. The needs of these patients are unique and nursing care demands great. For successful outcomes to be realized, nursing care assessment and interventional strategies must be tailored to this unique transplant population. Is intestine transplantation the short gut solution?

REFERENCES

Abu-Elmagd, K., Todo, S., Tzakis, A., Furukawa, H., Nour, B., Reyes, J., Nakamura, K., Scotti-Foglieni, C., El-Hammadi, H., Kadry, Z., Fung, J., Demetris, J., & Starzl, T.E. (1994). Rejection of human intestinal allografts: Alone or in combination with the liver. *Transplantation Proceedings, 26,* 1430–1431.

Cipriani, L., & Martin, S. (1994). Current controversies in pediatric transplantation. *AACN Clinical Issues in Critical Care, 5,* 263–277.

Funovits, M., Altieri, K. A., Kovalak, J. A., & Staschak-Chicko, S.M. (1993). Small intestine transplantation: A nursing perspective. *Critical Care Nursing Clinics of North America, 5,* 203–213.

Lillehei, R. C., Goott, B., & Miller, F. A. (1959). The physiologic response of the small bowel of the dog to ischemia including prolonged in vitro preservation of the bowel with successful replacement and survival. *Annals of Surgery, 150,* 543–560.

Reyes, J., Todo, S., Tzakis, A., Abu-Elmagd, K., Nour, B., Furukawa, H., & Starzl, T. E. (1994). Transplantation of the small bowel and other abdominal organs in humans. In L. S. Sher & L. Makowka (Eds.), *Intra-abdominal organ transplantation 2000* (pp. 165–181). Austin, TX: R.G. Landes.

Reyes, J., Tzakis, A. G., Scantlebury, V., Armitage, J., Nour, B., Green, M., Nalesnik, M., Yunis, E., Kauffman, M., Cipriani, L., Shapiro, R., & Michaels, M. (1994, August 28–31). Posttransplant lymphoproliferative disease after whole organ transplantation under FK506 immunosuppression in children. XVth World Congress of the Transplantation Society, Kyoto, Japan.

Reyes, J., Tzakis, A. G., Todo, S., Nour, B., & Starzl, T. E. (1993). Small bowel and liver/small bowel transplantation in children. *Seminars in Pediatric Surgery, 2,* 289–300.

Tzakis, A. G., Reyes, J., Nour, B., Marino, I. R., Todo, S., & Starzl, T. E. (1993). Temporary end-to-side portocaval shunt in orthotopic liver transplantation. *Journal of Surgery, Gynecology and Obstetrics, 176,* 181–182.

United Network for Organ Sharing. (1994 August). *UNOS Update, 10,* 38.

Weaver, L. T. (1991). Anatomy and embryology. In W. A. Walker, J. R. Hamilton, & J. A. Walker-Smith (Eds.), *Pediatric gastroenterology disease: Vol. I. Pathophysiology, diagnosis, management* (pp. 195–216). Philadelphia: B. C. Decker.

Wesson, D. (1991). The intestine: Part 1. Congenital anomalies. In W. A. Walker, J. R. Hamilton, & J. A. Walker-Smith (Eds.), *Pediatric gastroenterology disease: Vol. I. Pathophysiology, diagnosis, management* (pp. 477–484). Philadelphia: B. C. Decker.

16

ALTERNATIVES TO CARDIAC RETRANSPLANTATION

Helen Luikart, R.N., M.S.

Heart transplantation is a well-accepted therapy for end-stage heart disease. Current indications for transplantation are coronary artery disease, cardiomyopathy, valvular disease, and congenital heart defects. Current one-year actuarial survival is generally accepted as 82 to 85% for first transplant and less than 65% for retransplantation later than 6 months after the first (Hosenpud, Novick, Breen, & Daily, 1994). In 1993 there were 2,299 heart transplants and 72 retransplants performed in the United States (United Network for Organ Sharing [UNOS], 1994). The primary causes of death within the first 12 months are graft failure, rejection, and infection. After the first 12 months, the major cause of death is allograft coronary artery disease (ACAD), also referred to as accelerated graft atherosclerosis.

Retransplantation is currently the only therapy available to prevent death from ACAD (Schroeder et al., 1993). Due to the increasing numbers of heart transplants performed each year, there is a growing number of patients affected by ACAD. Clinicians are frequently faced with the dilemma to consider retransplant despite poor retransplant survival rates. Ethical dilemmas come to the forefront when considering allocation of limited donor hearts. While some consider retransplant the only viable option, other routes are being explored to optimize organ use (Schroeder et al., 1993). Percutaneous transluminal angioplasty, atherectomy, or coronary artery bypass grafting are potential alternatives for a limited number of patients with end-stage allograft coronary artery disease.

ALLOGRAFT CORONARY ARTERY DISEASE

Allograft coronary artery disease is not wholly understood in its etiology or progression. Some believe it to be chronic rejection because it may be an immunologic response at the site of the coronary artery endothelium (Copeland, Butman, & Gulshaw, 1990; Gao et al., 1989; Halle et al., 1992). Others believe ACAD may be due to injury during preservation or the combination of one or more of the known risk factors for native CAD (Copeland et al., 1990; Gao et al., 1989). Risk factors for retransplant have been identified. These factors include an increased number of treated rejection episodes, elevated cholesterol (especially LDL) (Gao, Schroeder, Hunt, & Stinson, 1988), hypertension, chronic prednisone therapy, positive cytomegalovirus serology, cigarette smoking, positive post-transplant antibodies, and donor hearts older than 40 years (see Table 16.1) (Halle et al., 1992).

Approximately 40 to 50% of patients have angiographic evidence of ACAD by 5 years post-transplant (Christensen, Meyer, Iacarella, Kubo, & Wilson, 1994; Halle et al., 1992; Schroeder et al., 1993). Once angiographic evidence of ACAD is present, patients are at greater risk for subsequent cardiac events (Uretsky et al., 1992).

Allograft coronary artery disease is diffuse in nature, usually involving mid- and terminal branches of major vessels (Copeland et al., 1990). This distal-vessel obliteration, referred to as pruning, is in contrast to native heart CAD, which exhibits distinct focal occlusions within the coronary artery. Transplant coronary disease may progress rapidly, unlike native heart CAD. Angiographic changes may be seen in as little as 6 months. Presenting symptoms may include a deterioration in ventricular function, congestive heart failure, ventricular arrhythmias, and sudden death (Halle et al., 1992). Anginal pain is uncommon due to heart denervation. Ischemic events may be silent and painless, and infarction can go undetected without regular evaluation (Vetrovec et al., 1988). Stark, McGinn and Wilson (1991) reported several cases of patients who appear to have cardiac reinnervation several years post-transplant. This was demonstrated

TABLE 16.1 Potential Risk Factors for Allograft Coronary Artery Disease

- History of hypertension
- History of treated acute rejection
- Chronic prednisone immunosuppression
- Positive CMV serology
- Cigarette smoking
- Serum cholesterol >300 mg/l
- Positive post-transplant antibodies
- Donor over 40 years of age

Sources: Adapted from "Retransplantation for severe accelerated coronary artery disease in heart transplant recipients," by S. Z. Gao, J. S. Schroeder, S. A. Hunt, & E. B. Stinson, 1988. *The American Journal of Cardiology, 62,* pp. 876–881. "Coronary angioplasty in cardiac transplant patients results of a multi-center study," by A. A. Halle, R. F. Wilson, E. K. Massin, R. C. Bourge, M. L. Stadius, M. R. Johnson, R. B. Wray, J. B. Young, R. A. Davies, G. D. Walford, L. W. Miller, U. Deligonul, G. Rincon, S. H. Kubo, G. DiSiascio, C. C. Crandall, M. J. Cowley, & G. W. Vetrovec, 1992, *Circulation, 86,* pp. 458–462.

in patient complaints of classic anginal pain in the face of known ACAD. Complaints of chest pain, therefore, should not be disregarded.

Most transplant centers evaluate heart recipients for the onset or progression of ACAD on an annual or semiannual basis. Heart transplant clinicians have been trying to develop noninvasive methods to identify the onset and progression of ACAD. Echocardiography, treadmill testing, gated-wall motion testing, Holter exercise, and thallium testing have all proven to have limited sensitivity in the detection of ACAD (Jain et al., 1993). Intravascular ultrasonography (IVUS) is an invasive imaging technique that provides characterization of vessel wall morphology by ultrasound imaging in the coronary arteries. Some transplant centers perform IVUS at the time of the annual coronary arteriogram. It is proving to be the most sensitive method to assess the presence and progress of ACAD (St. Goar et al., 1992).

ALLOGRAFT CORONARY ARTERY DISEASE MANAGEMENT

Currently there is no known prophylaxis for the prevention of ACAD and no medical therapy to arrest or even slow the progress of the disease (Mullins et al., 1991). Recent studies have shown a promising decrease in the incidence and time of onset of ACAD when calcium channel blockers are used immediately post-transplant (Schroeder et al., 1993). Actual progression of the disease is not amenable to treatment due to its diffuse nature.

Percutaneous Transluminal Angioplasty

Percutaneous transluminal coronary angioplasty (PTCA) is a widely accepted therapy for native CAD. Its safety and beneficial results are well documented (Christensen et al., 1994; Landau, Lange, & Hillis, 1994). In the transplanted heart, ACAD has been shown to be particularly severe in medium and small coronary arteries, usually involving the distal segment. A small number of transplant patients do present with focal stenosis in the large epicardial coronary arteries, appearing angiographically similar to native CAD. In these patients, PTCA has been used successfully (Christensen et al., 1994; Halle et al., 1992).

Primary indications for PTCA in the transplanted heart, in addition to discrete angiographic CAD, are evidence of silent ischemia and symptomatic ischemia such as exercise-induced dyspnea, rapidly progressive CAD, worsening congestive heart failure, or decreasing left ventricular function (see Table 16.2) (Halle et al., 1992; Sandhu et al., 1992).

Successful ballooning of a lesion has been defined as improvement in luminal patency of less than 50% occlusion, or an average of 46% reduction in stenosis, as well as a significant reduction in coronary pressure gradients pre- versus post-PTCA (Christensen et al., 1994; Halle et al., 1992; Mullins et al., 1991). Few complications have been noted. These complications were localized intimal dissection (Mullins et al., 1991) and ventricular fibrillation during PTCA due to spasm of the dilated artery. Ventricular fibrillation was treated with electrical cardioversion, and intracoronary nitroglycerin was used to treat vasospasm (Sandhu et al., 1992). Other complications reported include myocardial infarction with subsequent death 1 week after PTCA, groin hematomas, and exacerbation of renal insufficiency (Halle et al., 1992). Restenosis is a late complication that occurs in 25 to 50% of the patients less than one year after PTCA (Christensen et al., 1994; Halle et al., 1992). Restenosis is usually defined as an artery that has a return of 40 to 50% occlusion. Restenosis may be redilated without additional risk.

A major drawback to PTCA in the cardiac transplant patient is that, in the event of a major complication, surgical support for emergent coronary artery bypass surgery may have to be considered in spite of the high risk of surgery. Some patients may need intra-aortic balloon pump assistance as a bridge to retransplantation instead of bypass grafting (Halle et al., 1992).

PTCA in the transplant population is not procedurally different than in nontransplant patients. The standard over-the-wire technique is generally used. Arterial access is obtained via the femoral artery, and the catheter is advanced to the coronary ostium. Continuous intravenous nitroglycerin

TABLE 16.2 Primary Indications for PTCA in Transplant Patients

- Rapidly progressing ACAD
- Evidence of ischemia
- Symptomatic ischemia
- Worsening CHF
- Decreased left ventricular function
- Focal lesion(s)

Sources: Adapted from "Coronary angioplasty in cardiac transplant patients: results of a multi-center study," by A. A. Halle, R. F. Wilson, E. K. Massin, R. C. Bourge, M. L. Stadius, M. R. Johnson, R. B. Wray, J. B. Young, R. A. Davies, G. D. Walford, L. W. Miller, U. Deligonul, G. Rincon, S. H. Kubo, G. DiSiascio, C. C. Crandall, M. J. Cowley, & G. W. Vetrovec, 1992, *Circulation, 86,* pp. 458–462. "Potential limitations of percutaneous transluminal coronary angioplasty in heart transplant recipients," by J. S. Sandhu, B. F. Uretsky, S. Reddy, B. G. Denys, R. J. Ruffner, W. M. Breisblatt, T. R. Zerbe, R. L. Kormos, J. M. Armitage, R. L. Hardesty, & B. P. Griffith, 1992, *The American Journal of Cardiology, 69,* pp. 1234–1237.

infusion is used, and intravenous heparin is given by bolus to maintain an optimal clotting time. An angioplasty guidewire and balloon are advanced through the stenosis, and the lesion is dilated (Christensen et al., 1994).

Directional Coronary Atherectomy

Directional coronary atherectomy (DCA) is a relatively new procedure in the treatment of discrete atheromatous lesions. It is being considered as an alternative to PTCA for similar indications in the native and transplanted heart. The ideal candidate for this procedure is a patient with a localized eccentric lesion in a proximal to mid-coronary artery segment (Strikwerda et al., 1992). Advantages cited by researchers for DCA are the ability to debulk the atheromatous plaque and possibly decrease the incidence of restenosis (Jain et al., 1993). This procedure enables histologic analysis of removed tissue, which may contribute to further understanding of the pathogenesis of allograft coronary artery disease (Jain et al., 1993; Strikwerda et al., 1992). The benefits and long-term outcome of DCA compared to PTCA have not been assessed due to the small number of DCA procedures. Currently, it has not been associated with any increase in complications over PTCA (Jain et al., 1993; Strikwerda et al., 1992).

Post-PTCA or DCA nursing care is similar to that involved in nontransplant patients except that anginal pain is not generally seen in these patients; therefore, evaluation of heart rhythm and complex should be carefully monitored for acute dissection or thrombosis. The immunocompromised host should be assessed for the early onset of infection. Fevers should be reported and followed by appropriate infection surveillance.

Coronary Artery Bypass Grafting

Coronary artery bypass grafting (CABG) in the transplanted heart has been performed on a very limited number of patients. The application of this procedure is limited due to the diffuse nature of the ACAD, the associated poor runoff of the coronary vessels, and the poor condition of the patients (Dunning et al., 1992).

The primary indication for CABG is a discrete proximal coronary stenosis in the transplant patient who is unsuitable for retransplantation or too hemodynamically unstable to wait for a donor heart.

Chronic immunosuppression is a major mortality risk factor for CABG in transplant recipients. Steroids cause delay in wound healing and increase tissue friability, and immunosuppression increases the risk of infection (Copeland et al., 1990). Patients who have been on cyclosporine usually have some renal insufficiency, which is aggravated by the effects of general anesthesia and bypass time. The nephrotoxic effects of cyclosporine usually decrease patients' renal function over time so that any stressor such as hypotension may cause acute tubular necrosis. Many patients are obese post-transplant as a consequence of chronic steroid use. Obesity superimposed on the effects of steroids predisposes the patient to sternal infections (Dunning et al., 1992). Repeat sternotomy requires dissection of adhesions, which can prolong operating and bypass pump time, increasing the risk of bleeding complications. Repeat sternotomy may also limit the surgeons' ability to use the internal mammary artery for grafting, leaving only the saphenous veins for use (Dunning et al., 1992) (see Table 16.3).

Retransplantation

Retransplantation is a controversial procedure for the treatment of ACAD; however, it is the only known procedure that prolongs the survival of the patient (Schroeder et al., 1993). Retransplant occurs in 2.3% of all heart transplants done in the United States. The 1-year survival rate of patients undergoing retransplant less than 6 months after the original transplant is cited as 42% at one year versus a 64% one-year survival rate for those patients retransplanted greater than 6 months after the first transplant (Hosenpud et al., 1994). Retransplantation is indicated for patients with severe ACAD, intractable acute rejection, and restrictive and/or constrictive disease (Gao et al., 1988). Most patients retransplanted greater than 6 months after their first are retransplanted for ACAD.

Retransplant complications include perioperative bleeding, mediastinitis, and acute renal failure requiring dialysis (Ensley et al., 1992). Those patients surviving the operation and postoperative period show no dif-

TABLE 16.3 Risk Factors for Morbidity and Mortality post-CABG in the Transplant Recipient

- Chronic steroid use
- Chronic immunosuppression
- Repeat sternotomy
- Renal insufficiency
- Obesity

Sources: Adapted from "Successful coronary artery bypass grafting for high-risk left main coronary artery atherosclerosis after cardiac transplantation," by J. G. Copeland, S. M. Butman, & S. Gulshaw, 1990, *Annals of Thoracic Surgery, 49,* pp. 106–110. "Coronary artery bypass grafting nine years after cardiac transplant," by J. J. Dunning, S. W. H. Kendal, P. A. Mullins, A. Chauhan, T. R. Grahm, B. Biocina, P. M. Schofield, & S. R. Large, 1992, *Annals of Thoracic Surgery, 54,* pp. 571-572.

ference in long-term infection or rejection. However, a greater sensitivity to HLA antigens, a higher incidence of positive retrospective cross-match, and a higher incidence of nonskin malignancies were noted (Ensley et al., 1992). Long-term follow-up of these patients shows that they have a high incidence of recurrent ACAD (Gao et al., 1988).

ACAD Ethical Management

Ethical considerations abound due to the widespread shortage of donor organs. Because of limited donor availability, many transplant centers are questioning the allocation of organs to less than ideal candidates. The fairness of allocating organs to individuals for a second transplant is questioned when other people die while waiting for their first (Ubel, Arnold, & Caplan, 1993). The practice is particularly criticized when the outcome is known to be discouraging (Ensley et al., 1992). Conversely, many transplant centers in the United States offer their patients retransplantation because transplant physicians feel they have a commitment to patients and a duty not to abandon them with a failing graft (Ubel et al., 1993).

Currently, the system of donor allocation applies equally to retransplant candidates. Blood type and wait time prioritize listings; however, if a retransplant candidate is on life support, he or she can advance to a status 1 category and get priority over status 2 candidates.

SUMMARY

Allograft coronary artery disease is a major limiting factor in the long-term survival of cardiac transplant recipients. There is currently no known prevention or treatment for accelerated graft atherosclerosis. Much of the current research is aimed at understanding this form of chronic rejection. Some new immunosuppressant medications are thought to inhibit the development of ACAD, but long clinical trials place the medications years away from clinical use at this time.

Medical and/or surgical management are the only options for patients, and those are limited due to the diffuse nature of the disease. PTCA has been shown to be effective in the heart transplant recipient who demonstrates discrete proximal epicardial stenosis. While the success and complication rates have been reported comparable to those in nonheart transplant patients (Christensen et al., 1994; Halle et al., 1992), Sandhu et al. (1992) found that long-term outcome may not be good. This group concluded that confirmation of high-grade proximal disease yielded a low probability of long-term survival.

Coronary artery bypass grafting in a transplant allograft has been an effective method of therapy in a few select patients who meet strict criteria. Patients who are at risk for sudden death or serious cardiac dysfunction may benefit from CABG even if they are at high risk.

Retransplantation has proven to be the only life-prolonging treatment for ACAD. While results show that retransplantation has greater mortality than a first transplant, centers continue to see this risky and only moderately successful procedure as the only option to save their patients' lives. Children may have better results than adults, but the number of pediatric retransplants remains small. Retransplantation remains controversial because of the limited donor supply and the belief that the donor allografts should go to those who would benefit the most and to those who have the greatest chance of survival.

Alternatives to retransplantation offer a hopeful future for some patients with end-stage ACAD. Pharmaceutical breakthroughs and improved surgical and interventional techniques may one day offer patients and their clinicians greater choices in therapy. Ethics of organ allocation will always be at the heart of any debate regarding retransplantation and its alternatives.

REFERENCES

Christensen, B. V., Meyer, S. M., Iacarella, C. L., Kubo, S. H., & Wilson, R. W. (1994). Coronary angioplasty in heart transplant recipients: A quantitative angiographic long term follow-up study. *The Journal of Heart and Lung Transplantation, 13,* 212–220.

Copeland, J. G., Butman, S. M., & Gulshaw, S. (1990). Successful coronary artery bypass grafting for high-risk left main coronary artery atherosclerosis after cardiac transplantation. *Annals of Thoracic Surgery, 49,* 106–110.

Dunning, J. J., Kendal, S. W. H., Mullins, P. A., Chauhan, A., Grahm, T. R., Biocina, B., Schofield, P. M., & Large, S. R. (1992). Coronary artery bypass grafting nine years after cardiac transplant. *Annals of Thoracic Surgery, 54,* 571–572.

Ensley, R. D., Hunt, S. A., Taylor, D. O., Renlund, D. G., Menlove, R. L., Karawande, S. V., O'Connell, J. B., Barr, M. L., Michler, R. E., Copeland, J. G., & Miller, L. W. (1992). Predictors of survival after repeat heart transplantation. *The Journal of Heart and Lung Transplantation, 11,* S142–S158.

Gao, S. Z., Schroeder, J. S., Alderman, E. L., Hunt, S. A., Valantine, H. A., Wiederhold, V., & Stinson, E. B. (1989). Prevalence of accelerated coronary artery disease in heart transplant survivors. *Circulation, 3*(80) 100–105.

Gao, S. Z., Schroeder, J. S., Hunt, S. A., & Stinson, E. B. (1988). Retransplantation for severe accelerated coronary artery disease in heart transplant recipients. *The American Journal of Cardiology, 62,* 876–881.

Halle, A. A., Wilson, R. F., Massin, E. K., Bourge, R. C., Stadius, M. L., Johnson, M. R., Wray, R. B., Young, J. B., Davies, R. A., Walford, G. D., Miller, L. W., Deligonul, U., Rincon, G., Kubo, S. H., DiSiascio, G., Crandall, C. C., Cowley, M. J., & Vetrovec, G. W. (1992). Coronary angioplasty in cardiac transplant patients results of a multi-center study. *Circulation, 86,* 458–462.

Hosenpud, J. D., Novick, R. J., Breen, T. J., & Daily, O. P. (1994). The registry of the International Society of Heart and Lung Transplant: Eleventh official report: 1994. *The Journal of Heart and Lung Transplantation, 13,* 561–570.

Jain, S. P., Ventura, H. O., Ramee, S. R., Collins, T. J., Isner, J. M., & White, C. J. (1993). Directional coronary atherectomy in heart transplant recipients. *The Journal of Heart and Lung Transplantation, 12,* 819–823.

Landau, C., Lange, R. A., & Hillis, L. D. (1994). Percutaneous transluminal coronary angioplasty. *The New England Journal of Medicine, 330,* 981–993.

Mullins, P. A., Shapiro, L. M., Aravot, D. A., Scott, J. P., Large, S. R., Wallwork, J., & Schofield, P. M. (1991). Experience of percutaneous transluminal coronary angioplasty in orthotopic cardiac transplant recipients. *European Heart Journal, 12,* 1205–1207.

Sandhu, J. S., Uretsky, B. F., Reddy, S., Denys, B. G., Ruffner, R. J., Breisblatt, W. M., Zerbe, T. R., Kormos, R. L., Armitage, J. M., Hardesty, R. L., & Griffith, B. P. (1992). Potential limitations of percutaneous transluminal coronary angioplasty in heart transplant recipients. *The American Journal of Cardiology, 69,* 1234–1237.

Schroeder, J. S., Gao, S. Z., Alderman, E. L., Hunt, S. A., Johnstone, I., Boothroyd, D. B., Wiederhold, V., & Stinson, E. B. (1993). A preliminary study of diltiazem in the prevention of coronary artery disease in heart-transplant recipients. *New England Journal of Medicine, 328,* 164–170.

Stark, R. P., McGinn, A. L., & Wilson, R. F. (1991). Chest pain in cardiac transplant recipients: Evidence of sensory reinnervation after cardiac transplantation. *The New England Journal of Medicine, 324,* 1791–1794.

St. Goar, F. G., Pinto, F. J., Alderman, E. L., Valantine, H. V., Schroeder, J. S., Gao, S. Z., Stinson, E. B., & Popp, R. L. (1992). Intracoronary ultrasound in cardiac transplant recipients: In vivo evidence of "angiograghically silent" intimal thickening. *Circulation, 85,* 979–984.

Strikwerda, S., Umans, V., van der Linden, M. M., van Suylen, R. J., Balk, A. H., de Feyter, P. J., Serruys, P. W., & van Swijndregt, E. M. (1992). Percutaneous directional atherectomy for discrete coronary lesions in cardiac transplant patients. *American Heart Journal, 123,* 1686–1690.

Ubel, P. A., Arnold, R. M., & Caplan, A. L. (1993). Rationing failure: The ethical lessons of the retransplantation of scarce vital organs. *Journal of the American Medical Association, 270,* 2469–2474.

United Network for Organ Sharing (UNOS) (1994). *UNOS scientific registry: Appendix D-V: Heart recipients: 1988–1993.* Richmond, VA.

Uretsky, B. F., Kormos, R. L., Zerbe, T. R., Lee, A., Tokarczyk, T. R., Murali, S., Reddy, P. S., Denys, B. G., Griffith, B. P., Hardesty, R. L., Armitage, J. M., & Arena, V. C. (1992). Cardiac events after heart transplantation: Incidence and predictive value of coronary arteriography. *The Journal of Heart and Lung Transplantation, 11,* S45–S51.

Vetrovec, G. W., Cowley, M. J., Newton, C. M., Lewis, S. A., DiSciascio, G., Thompson, J. A., Hastill, W. A., Lower, R., & Hess, M. (1988). Applications of percutaneous transluminal coronary angioplasty in cardiac transplantation. *Circulation, 3,* 83–88.

17

AUTOLOGOUS BONE MARROW TRANSPLANT FOR BREAST CANCER

Angela Johns, R.N., M.P.A., O.C.N.

Breast cancer is the second leading cause of cancer deaths among women. In the United States, more than 180,000 women a year are diagnosed with breast cancer, and 46,000 women die annually of the disease. A great deal of debate exists among medical professionals regarding the most appropriate treatment. The controversy regarding treatment approaches for high-risk and advanced breast cancer is whether or not bone marrow transplantation provides a greater chance of cure than standard therapy. A number of clinical trials have demonstrated the efficacy of autologous bone marrow transplantation (ABMT) in generating complete response (CR) or partial response (PR) in advanced and high-risk breast cancer (Antman & Armitage, 1992; Antman & Gale, 1988). This chapter describes the different stages of breast cancer and discusses the option of bone marrow transplantation for Stages II, III, and IV disease. The risks and anticipated benefits of transplantation will also be reviewed. However, the answer to the question of whether high dose chemotherapy with autologous bone marrow support provides increased survival is yet to be determined by randomized clinical trials.

Bone marrow transplantation (BMT), a treatment modality that has been in use for the past 25 years, is increasingly used to treat aggressive cancers. The first malignancy treated with bone marrow transplantation was advanced leukemia refractory to standard chemotherapy. The initial results of the procedure were encouraging when a small percentage of patients with a uniformly fatal disease responded to this aggressive experimental therapy. BMT is now standard therapy for leukemia, aggressive lymphoma, and recurrent Hodgkin's disease because these types of malignant cells are chemotherapy and radiation therapy-responsive tumors. Evidence also exists to suggest that breast cancer cells are also chemotherapy-responsive.

STAGING AND STANDARD TREATMENT OF BREAST CANCER

Breast cancer is staged according to the size of the tumor and whether or not axillary lymph nodes contain malignant cells. (See Table 17.1 for complete listing of stages, prevalence, and prognosis.)

Carcinoma in Situ

This very early form of breast cancer accounts for 12% of newly diagnosed cases. Women with this disease, using standard therapy, have a 5-year survival rate of 95% (Weiss, 1994).

Stage I

Stage I breast cancer accounts for 38% of newly diagnosed cases. Women with this disease, using standard therapy, have a 5-year survival rate of 85%. Tumors less than 2 cm in size with no malignant cells in the axillary lymph nodes are characterized as Stage I. Breast cancer in situ and Stage I are treated with mastectomy, removal of the breast, or lumpectomy, removal of tumor, and surrounding tissue followed by local radiation therapy. The tumor is also tested to determine whether it has estrogen receptor sites on the malignant cell. If the receptor sites are present, the tumor is classified as estrogen receptor (ER) positive, and adjuvant hormonal treatment is started. Adjuvant therapy is initiated to assist in the control of the disease. Tamoxifen, an anti-estrogen agent, has been tested in large randomized studies and has proven effective in reducing recurrence rates in ER-positive women (Harris, Morrow, & Bonadonna, 1993).

TABLE 17.1 Cancer Stages and Prognosis

Stage	% of New Cases	5-Year Survival Rate
In situ	12%	>95%
Stage I	38%	85%
Stage II	31%	66%
Stage III	5.1%	41%
Stage IV	4.4%	10%

Source: Adapted from "Breast Cancer," by R. Weiss, 1994, April 19, *Washington Post*, pp. 14–15.

Bone marrow transplantation is not indicated for women with carcinoma in situ or Stage I disease.

Stage II

Stage II breast cancer is characterized by a tumor that is 2 to 5 cm in size, with or without positive lymph nodes. The status of lymph node involvement is an important indicator of prognosis. Common sites of regional lymph node involvement with tumor cells include the axillary, internal mammary, and supraclavicular nodes. The axillary lymph nodes are the most frequent sites of regional spread of malignant cells. Approximately 40% of women with breast cancer have axillary nodal involvement of the disease (Harris et al., 1993). Tumors larger than 5 cm without positive lymph nodes are also considered Stage II.

The size of tumor and the number of positive lymph nodes significantly influence the recurrence rate and the overall prognosis. Recurrence rates over a 5-year period range from 8 to 13% for women with tumors less than 2 cm without axillary nodal involvement. Women with tumors from 2 to 5 cm in size without nodal involvement have a recurrence rate of 19 to 24%. Women with tumors greater than 5 cm without nodal involvement have a 5-year recurrence rate of 19 to 27% (Weiss, 1994).

Axillary lymph nodes that test positive for malignant cells increase the recurrence rate in all breast tumors regardless of size. Tumors less than 2 cm in diameter with positive lymph nodes have a relapse rate of 37 to 50%. Tumors ranging from 2 to 5 cm with positive lymph nodes have a recurrence rate of 50 to 64%. Tumors larger than 5 cm have a recurrence rate of 65 to 79%.

Stage III

Stage III breast cancer is characterized by a tumor larger than 5 cm with positive axillary lymph nodes. The 5-year survival rate for women with

Stage III breast cancer is 41%. Researchers are actively involved in working on treatment plans to reduce recurrence rates in Stage II and Stage III breast cancer patients. Standard treatment includes surgical removal of the tumor and adjacent tissue with lymph node biopsies. Either a modified radical mastectomy or a breast-conserving lumpectomy with local radiation therapy can be performed. Each approach has an equal survival rate (Harris et al., 1993).

Adjuvant chemotherapy for Stage II and Stage III breast cancer is instituted to reduce the risk of recurrence from systemic spread of tumor cells. The standard approach includes multiple cycles of combination chemotherapy including cyclophosphamide, methotrexate, and fluorouracil (CMF). Doxorubicin has been substituted for methotrexate (CAF) in some studies.

Stage IV

Stage IV, or metastatic breast cancer, is characterized by a tumor of any size with evidence of distant disease at time of diagnosis. Frequent sites for metastatic disease include the liver, lung, or bone. The 5-year survival rate for metastatic breast cancer is 10%. The use of standard chemotherapy for metastatic breast cancer produces uniformly disappointing results. Complete remission rates range between 10% and 20% with the duration of remission limited to less than 16 months. The median rate of survival after diagnosis is 1 to 2 years. Standard chemotherapy provides no curative potential (Antman & Armitage, 1992; Antman & Gale, 1988).

HIGH DOSE CHEMOTHERAPY

The rationale for high dose chemotherapy and autologous bone marrow or stem cell support in breast cancer is the concept of dose intensity. Dose intensification enhances the tumor kill by delivering the maximum tolerated dose of chemotherapy. Without a bone marrow transplant, myelosuppression is a dose-limiting toxicity. Higher doses of chemotherapy can be administered when the marrow aplasia is rescued with autologous marrow or peripheral stem cell support. The approach to bone marrow transplant for breast cancer includes the following:

- choosing chemotherapy agents that are active against breast cancer cells in standard doses

- selecting a combination of chemotherapy agents with different organ-limiting toxicities
- administering the maximum tolerated dose

Other dose-limiting toxicities include cardiac, renal, hepatic, pulmonary, and mucositis. The use of autologous bone marrow transplant (ABMT) for Stage II and Stage III breast cancer is the center of debate between oncologists and transplant physicians. Randomized multicenter trials are under way to determine the effectiveness of ABMT in comparison to standard chemotherapy.

A number of transplant physicians are encouraged by studies that demonstrate a greater response rate with bone marrow transplantation than with standard chemotherapy for women with high-risk primary breast cancer. High-risk primary breast cancer is characterized by tumors greater than 2 cm with 10 or more positive nodes. Dr. Peters at Duke University reported a 72% event-free survival at a median follow-up of 2½ years after high dose chemotherapy and autologous bone marrow support (Peters et al., 1993). Historical controls showed event-free survival rates between 38% and 52% at 2½ years after standard adjuvant chemotherapy. Dr. Saez and colleagues studied breast cancer patients with 10 or more positive nodes at the University of Oklahoma and Tulsa Medical Center and found that after high dose chemotherapy and ABMT, 98% of the patients remain disease-free, with a median follow-up of 14 months (Saez, Selby, Strnadi, & Confer, 1993). Dr. Razis and colleagues found similar results at the New York Medical College (Razis et al., 1993). The initial results of these studies are encouraging, but we need to have a longer follow-up to determine if the response is durable.

ABMT for metastatic breast cancer has increased the number of patients who achieve a complete response and has increased the duration of the response. A study conducted at Indiana University using two cycles of high dose chemotherapy with ABMT has resulted in 43% of the patients alive and progression-free at a median time of 18 months. Dr. Williams and colleagues at the University of Chicago studied 59 patients with newly diagnosed breast cancer. After receiving high dose chemotherapy and bone marrow rescue, the median survival was 13⅓ months. The study concluded that ABMT has led to increased complete response rates, but the role of ABMT needs further refinement (Williams, Gilewski, Mick, & Biltran, 1992). In contrast, Dr. Peters reported encouraging results indicating that the overall response rate is 90% and 30% of metastatic patients alive and in complete remission at 3 years (Peters et al., 1993).

Recently, Dr. Long and colleagues at Stanford University have developed a repetitive-cycle combination chemotherapy protocol for women with metastatic breast cancer. This approach includes high-dose etoposide for stem cell mobilization and apheresis followed by four cycles of mitaxantrone, thiotepa, taxol, and cyclophosphamide. After each cycle, the patient receives 25% of the collected stem cells. The chemotherapy is administered in the outpatient setting with daily clinic and home care visits. It is still too early to determine the effectiveness of this approach in treating metastatic breast cancer. This study has demonstrated that significant increases in dose can be accomplished with minimal toxicities and safely administered in the outpatient setting.

AUTOLOGOUS BMT

While bone marrow transplantation remains controversial, according to the North American Autologous Bone Marrow Transplant Registry, the number of women receiving transplantation for breast cancer in North America has increased from 258 in 1989 to 873 in 1992 (Antman, Rowlings, Armitage, & Horowitz, 1995). The transplant procedure is complex and requires a strong patient commitment and financial support. The patient is evaluated by the medical team to be sure she can tolerate the high dose chemotherapy. A thorough physical examination and laboratory testing of renal and hepatic function are performed prior to acceptance as a BMT candidate. Cardiac and pulmonary functions are also assessed to be sure the heart and lungs are not impaired from previous chemotherapy or coexisting diseases. After the patient has been cleared as an appropriate candidate, the patient is then fully informed of the risks and potential benefits of this aggressive treatment plan. Informed consent is then obtained from the patient before the process starts.

Autologous BMT Procedure

BMT is a five-phase process, including:

- harvesting
- conditioning
- infusion of marrow/transplant
- isolation/neutropenia
- recovery

Harvesting. The patient's marrow is harvested in the operating room under anesthesia, then cryopreserved and stored until the patient has received the conditioning regimen. Peripheral stem cells are frequently collected in addition to or instead of bone marrow. Peripheral stem cells are collected by a process called apheresis. The patient is connected to an apheresis machine via a central catheter or a large vein. The blood is circulated through the apheresis machine, and the mononuclear cells are removed while the blood and plasma are returned to the patient. The apheresis product is then processed in the BMT laboratory and cryopreserved until ready for infusion.

Conditioning. The conditioning regimen, which includes several days of high dose chemotherapy, is the second phase of treatment. The goal of the conditioning regimen is to eliminate the malignant cells with the use of combination chemotherapy and to prepare space within the bone for the previously harvested marrow. The high dose chemotherapy also eliminates the hematopoietic cells in the marrow, killing the remaining marrow. The patient must then be rescued with the previously harvested bone marrow or peripheral mononuclear cells to reconstitute her hematopoietic system.

Infusion of Marrow/Transplant. The third phase of transplantation is the infusion of the bone marrow. The marrow infusion process is usually without incident and frequently anticlimactic. The marrow or peripheral stem cells are thawed at the bedside and immediately infused through a central vein catheter. The patient is premedicated with hydrocortisone and diphenhydramine to reduce the risk of reacting to the preservative dimethyl sulfoxide (DMSO). Nausea, chest tightness, and chills are not uncommon reactions and are usually limited to the time of infusion. Each bag of marrow or peripheral mononuclear cells is infused in less than 5 minutes.

Isolation/Neutropenia. The fourth phase of bone marrow transplantation is the neutropenic period. The absolute neutrophil count is less than 500 and frequently less that 100. The bone marrow is not producing white cells, red cells, or platelets. During this phase, the patient is placed in strict isolation to reduce the risk of infection. Red blood cells and platelets are infused to prevent hemorrhage and anemia. The neutropenic phase lasts from 10 to 14 days.

Recovery. The final phase of bone marrow transplantation is the recovery period. During this time, the patient's white cell count returns to normal, and the side effects of chemotherapy and neutropenia resolve. This process takes from several weeks to several months and varies widely between patients.

NURSING MANAGEMENT

During Harvesting

The care of patients after bone marrow harvest includes management of the side effects of general anesthesia, establishing pain control, and observing for signs of excessive bleeding. The patient usually is in the hospital for only one night and recovers quickly from the procedure.

If the patient is to have peripheral stem cells harvested, the nursing care is more complex. Prior to harvesting peripheral blood cells, the patient may receive high dose chemotherapy to drive stem cells from the marrow into the peripheral blood. This process is called stem cell mobilization. After a single dose of chemotherapy, the patient is discharged from the hospital and placed on growth factors to help stimulate the production of neutrophils. The nurse is responsible for teaching the patient to self-inject subcutaneously with the growth factor. The patient is also instructed in the care of a central catheter and how to reduce infectious risks during the period of neutropenia. When the absolute neutrophil count returns to greater than 1,000, the patient is apheresed for 2 to 3 days. Each apheresis procedure takes 3 to 4 hours per day.

During Conditioning

During the time the patient is receiving conditioning chemotherapy, the nursing care emphasis is on managing the side effects and providing patient education and support. The major side effects include nausea, vomiting, and diarrhea. Adequate control of gastrointestinal symptoms can usually be controlled with serotonin inhibitors, hypnotics, and benzodiazepines. Adequate hydration must be maintained to reduce the risk of renal failure and hemorrhagic cystitis. Anorexia and nausea are side effects that may impact the patient's ability to eat. Total parenteral nutrition is frequently added to supplement caloric intake. The conditioning phase lasts from 4 to 6 days depending on the protocol.

During Transplant

The day of transplant is usually quite exciting for the patient and family. There is rarely a problem with the reinfusion of marrow or stem cells. The entire process takes less than an hour, and the procedure is performed at the bedside by the physician or the nurse. Nursing care involves providing symptomatic relief for the limited side effects and providing support and enthusiasm for the process.

During Isolation

Neutropenia. The immediate post-transplant isolation phase holds the greatest risk for complications and side effects of treatment. Medical and nursing care plans address minimizing risk of serious complications and controlling side effects.

Infection Control. Patient education consists of instructing the patient to adopt infection-control measures designed to reduce the risk of infection from normal body flora and outside sources. The high dose chemotherapy affects the rapidly dividing cells in the mucous membranes of the mouth and gastrointestinal tracts. This disruption in the mouth and gastrointestinal system can allow for a portal of entry for bacterial flora or fungal organisms. Microbial seeding from the mouth is a significant infectious risk during the period of neutropenia. The patient is instructed to perform mouth care at least six times a day to reduce the risk of bacterial or fungal infections. Daily showers with antibacterial soap and meticulous perianal care are encouraged to reduce the risk of skin and gastrointestinal organisms entering the blood stream. Central lines are changed every 48 hours, and dressings are changed daily. Scrupulous hand washing is mandatory for all staff and visitors who come in contact with patients during the neutropenic phase. The patient is usually restricted to an isolation room that includes an air filtration system that reduces bacteria and fungal spores. The medical management during the neutropenic phase includes broad spectrum antibacterial and antifungal prophylaxis and monitoring laboratory values that reflect hepatic, pulmonary, and renal function. The neutropenic phase lasts from 1 to 2 weeks. The following are examples of mucositis and skin care protocols.

Mucositis Protocol

- Rinse mouth with normal saline and baking soda to remove debris.
- Gently clean mouth with toothette moistened with baking soda solution.
- Rinse oral cavity with antibacterial solution to reduce bacterial flora.
- Use antifungal topical medication to reduce risk of oral thrush.

Skin Care

- Shower daily with antibacterial soap.
- Change dressings daily around indwelling catheter site.
- Meticulously cleanse perianal area with soft disposable cloth and antimicrobial soap.
- Apply skin creams that contain soothing emollients without perfume or alcohol.

Bleeding. Thrombocytopenia, with platelet counts less than 10,000, is common after high dose chemotherapy. Bleeding precautions include prevention from injury, observation of the skin for petechia, and monitoring body fluids for signs of bleeding. When high-dose cyclophosphamide is used as part of the conditioning regimen, bladder irrigation is initiated to reduce the risk of hemorrhagic cystitis. Close observation and testing of urine, stool, and emesis are important nursing interventions for early detection of bleeding. Blood and platelets are transfused as indicated by physician order and patient condition until hematopoietic reconstitution occurs. Platelet and red cell engraftment usually take longer than white cell engraftment. Blood- and platelets-transfusion requirements frequently continue into the outpatient recovery phase.

Side Effect Management. The side effects associated with high dose chemotherapy and neutropenia can be distressing, but are usually self-limiting. The most common side effects include mucositis, skin changes, hair loss, delayed nausea, vomiting, and diarrhea. Nursing measures focus upon the relief or minimization of distress. Narcotic analgesics are initiated to control mouth and throat pain. Skin creams are applied to provide lubrication and protection to open areas. Antiemetic and antidiarrheal agents are administered to treat gastrointestinal symptoms. The side effects resolve as the white count returns and healing takes place. Hair loss is temporary, and hair will usually return within 6 months.

During Recovery

The fifth phase, or recovery period, begins when the absolute neutrophil count reaches 500. The return of the white count is the first sign of engraftment and the beginning of the healing process. The side effects begin to resolve, and the patient's need for antibiotics and nutrition support is eliminated. When the patient can consume adequate calories and is afebrile off antibiotics, he/she is ready for discharge from the hospital.

The hospital recovery phase can be anywhere from a couple of days to several weeks, depending on the extent of the side effects. After discharge, the healing process continues for 6 months to a year.

SERIOUS COMPLICATIONS ASSOCIATED WITH ABMT

Major complications that can occur during the transplant process include organ toxicities and infectious complications.

Pulmonary. Pulmonary toxicities include interstitial pneumonitis or diffuse alveolar hemorrhage. Interstitial pneumonitis is caused by chemotherapy-induced interstitial changes that interfere with oxygenation. Interstitial pulmonary changes can occur as an early complication or a late sequela. Treatment includes supplemental-oxygen and high-dose steroid therapies. Diffuse alveolar hemorrhage (DAH) is a complication of transplantation characterized by diffuse pulmonary bleeding and is diagnosed by bronchoalveolar lavage. The treatment for DAH includes high-dose steroid treatment and platelet support. Both of these pulmonary complications can be resolved if early and adequate treatment is instituted.

Hepatic. Veno-occlusive disease (VOD) is a serious hepatic complication that can occur as a result of high dose chemotherapy. Veno-occlusive disease is characterized by abnormal weight gain, right upper quadrant pain, and ascites. The hepatic veins become narrowed with microemboli, and hepatic congestion occurs. Ascites occurs due to partial vein congestion and subsequent leakage of fluid into the abdominal cavity. The medical approach to managing VOD is mainly prophylactic. Close monitoring of fluid balance and low-dose heparin therapy are two methods of reducing the risk of hepatic congestion. If liver disease develops, measures are taken to minimize the use of hepatotoxic agents, including parenteral nutrients and drugs metabolized by the liver. Efforts are made to establish fluid balance and maintain hemodynamic stability. Diuretics and dopamine are used to maintain adequate urine output and to protect renal function. Veno-occlusive disease remains a major clinical challenge that has a significant associated mortality.

Cardiac. Cardiac toxicity can also occur. Chemotherapy-induced myocardial changes can result in cardiomyopathy. Cardiomyopathy can result in reduced cardiac output and congestive heart failure. Standard treatment for cardiomyopathy, including inotropes, diuretics, and oxygen therapy, can be instituted. The damage to the myocardium can range from a mild reduction in ejection fraction without symptoms to severe debilitating cardiomyopathy.

SOCIAL AND ECONOMIC ISSUES

Support and encouragement are important aspects of nursing care during the entire transplant process. Aggressive treatment options for women with breast cancer are frightening. The fear of death during the procedure and the risk of relapse are the significant concerns expressed by these women. The transplant process takes several weeks or months, during which time the patient's life is severely disrupted. Patients and families may need to relocate closer to the transplant center. Relocation has a significant financial impact on the patient and family. Loss of work and the additional expense associated with relocation can create a major financial burden on the patient. Social workers play an important role in providing solutions for the housing and the economic support necessary for the transplant process.

Despite the risk of serious toxicities, expense, and uncertain results, many women are selecting ABMT as the treatment alternative for high-risk breast cancer. The long-term effectiveness of high dose chemotherapy with autologous bone marrow and stem cell support for high-risk and advanced breast cancer is the center of debate between health care providers and insurance companies.

The high cost of transplantation and the number of potential candidates for this expensive procedure has resulted in insurance company denials for bone marrow transplants. The majority of third-party payors consider transplantation for breast cancer as experimental and therefore exclude coverage. A number of women have successfully sued their insurance companies. As a result of these lawsuits and increasing public pressure, several insurance companies have agreed to pay for transplants if they are conducted as part of a randomized clinical trial (Chase, 1994).

Blue Cross/Blue Shield, the nation's largest health insurer, has agreed to support clinical trials sponsored by the National Cancer Institute (NCI) (The Blue Cross and Blue Shield, 1994). The clinical trials include high dose therapy for Stage II and Stage III breast cancer with 10 or more positive nodes or metastatic breast cancer. The clinical trials are multicenter, randomized trials comparing conventional chemotherapy to high dose chemotherapy with ABMT for the treatment of high-risk or advanced breast cancer. The NCI is coordinating three trials at more than 40 leading medical centers around the country. The results of these trials will not be available until 1999. At this point, no conclusions can be made about the effectiveness of high dose chemotherapy with autologous bone marrow transplants.

SUMMARY

Dr. Eddy at the Center for Health Policy, Research, and Education at Duke University reviewed studies to demonstrate evidence of the effectiveness of ABMT in the treatment of metastatic breast cancer. Dr. Eddy determined that firm conclusions were not possible due to the lack of randomized, controlled trials comparing standard therapy to high dose therapy (Eddy, 1992).

High-risk and advanced breast cancer continues to be a major medical challenge. Researchers are actively pursuing therapies that can provide long-term, disease-free survival. Autologous bone marrow transplantation holds some hope for treating these aggressive cancers, but there are significant costs and morbidity associated with this approach. The results of the national multicenter trials will help to answer the question of the most effective therapy to reduce the mortality associated with breast cancer.

REFERENCES

Antman, K. H., & Armitage, J. O. (1992). Dose intensive therapy in breast cancer. In J. O. Armitage (Ed.), *High dose cancer therapy* (pp. 701–716). Baltimore: Williams and Wilkins.

Antman, K. H., & Gale, R. P. (1988). Advanced breast cancer: High dose chemotherapy and bone marrow autotransplants. *Annals of Internal Medicine, 108,* 570–574.

Antman, K. H., Rowlings, Armitage, J. O., & Horowitz, M. A. (1995). Autotransplant for breast cancer in North America. Data from the American Blood and Transplant Registry. *Proceedings of the American Society of Clinical Oncology.*

The Blue Cross and Blue Shield Demonstration Project on Breast Cancer, 1994 (a pamphlet).

Chase, M. (1994, February 17). Breast cancer patients seeking new therapy face tough obstacles. *Wall Street Journal,* p. 1.

Eddy, D. M. (1992). High dose chemotherapy with autologous bone marrow transplantation for the treatment of metastatic breast cancer. *Journal of Clinical Oncology, 10,* 657–670.

Harris, J. R., Morrow, M., & Bonadonna, G. (1993). Cancer of the breast. In V. T. DeVito (Ed.), *Cancer: Principles and practice of oncology* (4th ed., pp. 1264–1324). Philadelphia: J. B. Lippincott.

Peters, W. P., Ross, M., Vredenburgh, J. J., Meisenberg, B., Marks, L. M., Winer, E., Kurtzberg, J., Bast, R. C., Jones, R., Shpall, E., We, K., Rosner, G., Gilbert, C., Mathias, B., Coniglo, D., Petross, W., Hendeson, I. C., Norton, L., Weiss, R. B., Buchman, D., & Hurd, D. (1993). High dose chemotherapy and autologous bone marrow support as consolidation after standard dose adjuvant therapy for high-risk primary breast cancer. *Journal of Clinical Oncology, 11,* 1132–1143.

Razis, E., Moet, P., Cook, P., Mittleman, A., Chum, H. G., Moorhty, L., Helson, L., Puccio, C., Brady, J., Meese, T., Samonis, G., & Ahmed, T. (1993). Adjuvant chemotherapy for high risk stage II breast cancer with high dose thiotepa (T) mitoxantrone (M) and caroboplatunum (J) and autologous bone marrow support. *Proceedings of the American Society of Clinical Oncology, 12,* 103.

Saez, R. A., Selby, G. B., Strnadi, C. M., & Confer, D. L. (1993). High dose carpoplatin, etoposide and cyclophosphamide with autologous bone marrow transplantation (ABMT) for high risk stage II/III breast cancer. *Proceedings of the American Society of Clinical Oncology, 12,* 99.

Weiss, R. (1994, April 19). Breast cancer. *Washington Post Health,* pp. 14–15.

Williams, S. F., Gilewski, T., Mick, R., & Biltran, J. D. (1992). High-dose consolidation therapy with autologous stem-cell rescue in stage IV breast cancer: Follow-up report. *Journal of Clinical Oncology, 10,* 1743–1747.

INDEX